Saunders
Medical
Assisting
Pocket Pal

Saunders Medical Assisting Pocket Pal

Sue A. Hunt, MA, RN, CMA

Professor and Coordinator
Medical Assisting Program
Middlesex Community College
Lowell, Massachusetts

Contributing Writer:
Jon H. Zonderman
Orange, Connecticut

SAUNDERS
An Imprint of Elsevier

SAUNDERS

An Imprint of Elsevier

The Curtis Center
Independence Square West
Philadelphia, Pennsylvania 19106-3399

Editor-in-Chief: Andrew Allen
Senior Acquisitions Editor: Adrianne Williams
Senior Developmental Editor: Rae A. Robertson
Editorial Assistant: Elizabeth Melchor

Library of Congress Cataloging-in-Publication Data

Hunt, Sue A.
    Saunders medical assisting pocket pal / Sue A. Hunt ;
    contributing writer, Jon H. Zonderman.
       p. ; cm.
    Includes bibliographical references and index.
    ISBN 0-7216-9225-7
    1. Medical assistants—Handbooks, manuals, etc. 2. Clinical
competence—Handbooks, manuals, etc. 3. Medical offices—
Management—Handbooks, manuals, etc. I. Zonderman, Jon.
II. Title.
    [DNLM: 1. Allied Health Personnel—Handbooks. 2. Clinical
Competence—Handbooks. 3. Efficiency, Organizational—
Handbooks. 4. Forms and Records Control—organization &
administration—Handbooks. W 49 H943m 2002]
    R728.8 .H86 2002
    651'.961—dc21   2002021031

Permissions may be sought directly from Elsevier's Health Sciences Rights
Department in Philadelphia, USA: phone: (+1)215-238-7869, fax: (+1)215-238-2239,
email: healthpermissions@elsevier.com. You may also complete your request on-line
via the Elsevier Science homepage (http://www.elsevier.com), by selecting 'Customer
Support' and then 'Obtaining Permissions'.

Printed in the United States of America

Last digit is the print number: 9   8   7   6   5   4   3

Preface

The *Saunders Medical Assisting Pocket Pal* is designed to ease the transition from student to professional medical assistant. It can be used for reference both during the medical assisting externship and on the job. It will provide a pocket-size reference for procedures and important information that has been learned in the classroom, as well as a planner and notebook to keep track of information gathered in the early days of an externship or new job.

When beginning an externship or a new job, there is so much to remember. The *Pocket Pal* begins with tools for recording personal information related to the office or clinic where the medical assistant is doing his or her externship or beginning a new job. This part of the book includes:

- A section with pages to record telephone numbers, doctor preferences, useful web sites, goals, and objectives.
- A six-month calendar that can be used to keep track of hours scheduled and hours completed.
- Check-off sheets to record procedures completed under supervision and independently arranged according to the entry-level competencies of the American Association of Medical Assistants (AAMA).

The remainder of the book contains useful information for the medical assistant. Working in a medical office is different from being in a classroom or assisting in a medical lab, and the new medical assistant often needs to refresh his or her memory before performing procedures or activities that involve real patients. The information in this section is arranged in the order of the AAMA entry-level competencies, with an administrative section, a clinical section, and a section for the transdisciplinary competencies of communication, legal concepts, patient instruction, and operational functions. Drawings and photographs are used for visual reinforcement. Tables and boxes summarize important information.

This *Pocket Pal* is not intended to replace the medical assisting textbook that the student has used in class. The information it contains has been summarized from *Saunders Fundamentals of Medical Assisting,* but its convenient arrangement allows it to be used easily, no matter what textbook the student has used in class. Students can use the *Pocket Pal* to jog their memory, but they may need to refer to their textbook for a more complete review of information or procedures.

This compact book should be both a reference and a personal record during the stressful early days of an externship or new job. Personalize it, and use it often to help reduce stress and increase confidence as you make the transition from student to seasoned professional.

Sue A. Hunt, MA, RN, CMA

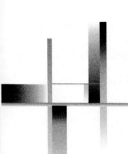

Contents

Preparing for Externship or New Job

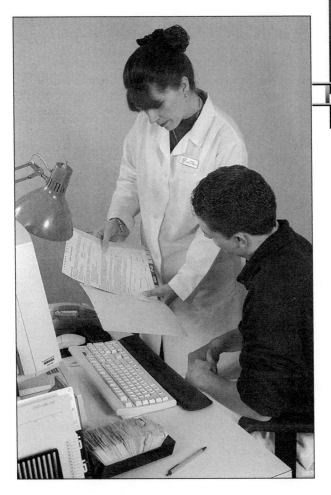

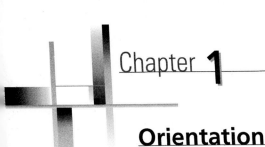

Chapter 1

Orientation

Working in a medical office as a medical assistant is a challenging adventure that will demand concentration and energy. You may be beginning the externship associated with your educational program, in which case you will be facing many new experiences. You will be carrying out procedures with patients that you have performed only in a classroom setting, and you will have responsibilities that you have never experienced before. Or you may be beginning your first job as a medical assistant. In this case there will also be many new responsibilities and experiences waiting for you.

KEYS TO A SUCCESSFUL EXPERIENCE

There are seven keys for making the externship or a new job a successful experience:

1. **Be on time and attend regularly.**
   The medical office relies on its personnel. Poor attendance or tardiness, especially early in the experience, is a message that you may be undependable.
2. **Present a professional appearance.**
   A clean, unwrinkled uniform with spotless shoes and tidy hair make you look competent and inspire trust and confidence in patients.
3. **Respond positively to any feedback.**
   In the beginning you are learning how things are done and how you can fit into this particular setting. Try to respond positively to any feedback, and do not take critiques of your behavior personally. Write down information you need to remem-

ber, and demonstrate that you are learning from what you are being told.

4. **Stay busy.**

Once the office is confident of your abilities to perform certain tasks, do them without being asked. Work to become a contributing team member who understands what needs to be done and pitches in to help others.

5. **Take time and care in your work.**

You may not be excited about every task you are asked to perform, but take care to do it accurately and avoid cutting corners. If you are blamed for mistakes, remember that the most recent addition to an office is often identified by staff members who have been there for a long time as the person most likely to have made an error. If this happens, don't take it personally; offer to try to help fix the mistake.

6. **Do not overstep your role.**

Be sure you understand what you are expected to do, and what the office staff want to check you off on before you perform independently. If you believe you are not being allowed to do enough, consider the possibility that staff members do not think they can depend on you or that you are not motivated. Ask for help if you are uncertain about a particular procedure, but if possible try to figure things out on your own.

7. **Do not gossip.**

Avoid the temptation to talk about personal issues or to become involved in conversations about employees or patients. If you have issues with staff members, either speak to them directly or speak to your supervisor or to your instructor if you are on externship. One of the challenges in any new work situation is to learn to deal with many individuals in a constructive way and to work out problems without falling into the unproductive cycle of complaining about situations instead of trying to change them.

ORIENTATION TO THE FACILITY

Your first responsibility is to become familiar with the medical office, clinic, or other medical setting where you will be working. You will probably be given a tour and introduced to many of the employees. On your first day you should write down the telephone number and extension of the person you must notify if you are delayed or must be absent. Do so on page 10 in the section for recording important telephone numbers. You may also want to record the names of employees and physicians. For many people, writing names is a helpful way to learn them. Table 1–1 summarizes the information that you should gather during the first week at the facility.

Avoid asking too many questions at once, but do ask enough

TABLE 1–1
Orientation to the Medical Office

Meet the Personnel
- Contact person or supervisor—record office telephone number and your supervisor's extension
- Person with whom you will work directly during orientation—record name and extension
- Physicians—record names if you have not already done so
- Other personnel who work in the office—record names if possible

Tour the Office
- Learn which exam rooms are used by each physician.
- Find out where you can leave your coat, purse, and personal belongings.
- Explore the layout of the front desk, exam rooms, supply rooms, the laboratory, the medical record area, and other areas in the office.
- Locate emergency equipment and emergency exits, including fire alarms, fire extinguishers, crash cart or emergency box, and emergency telephone numbers.
- When you are assigned to work in a specific area, locate supplies and equipment you will need to work effectively. For example, if you are sitting at the front desk, find pens and message forms. Become familiar with the telephone system found in your facility.

Identify Your Responsibilities
- Find out how you will know what to do each day, who will be working with you, and whom you should report to.
- Find out how to keep track of your hours or clock in and out. Determine exactly what your schedule will be. Find out when lunches and breaks are taken and how long they last.
- Identify the procedure for checking you off so that you can perform procedures independently.
- Find out what you are supposed to do if you have completed a task and there is no one available to show you something new.
- Find out if you are supposed to answer the telephone and, if so, what you should say as a greeting.
- Learn to work the intercom system. Learn how to let each physician know that a patient is waiting.

questions to become confident that you know what is expected of you and how to complete the tasks you have been assigned. Be sure to identify those individuals who like to help and to teach, since they are most approachable.

REVIEWING SKILLS

It is normal to feel concerned and a little anxious when you are asked to perform tasks involving real patients for the first time, especially when accuracy and proper technique are essential to provide care for the patient or when there is a possibility of hurting or injuring the patient. One way to increase confidence is to review the task or procedure before approaching the patient and, if possible, to mentally go through the steps. Use the second section of this book as a resource for review, as well as the office procedure manual, a drug reference to review any medications you may be asked to prepare or give, insurance and coding manuals, and other office reference materials. If you are shadowing an experienced medical assistant, observe how he or she carries out each task before attempting it yourself. You may also ask to perform skills such as vital signs on an office employee as a review before working with patients.

Observe how office staff document information and what kinds of teaching they do for patients. Clarify the kinds of information you can write in the patient's medical record as well as the kinds of information you are expected to give to patients, and locate any printed information that you can give to patients.

Look up any medication before preparing or giving it. Verify the spelling of medications you document in the chart using a drug reference. It takes time to learn the names of commonly used medications as well as their usual doses, side effects, and instructions you must give to the patient. You should prepare a medication card for any medication you have not given before as a tool to help you learn. *If you are allowed to give medication, you are legally liable for administering it properly to avoid harm to the patient.*

WORK ORGANIZATION

Take time before beginning work to identify your personal priorities each day and to organize your work day. If you are at an externship, you should write down objectives for each day using the sheets provided in

Chapter 2. At the end of the day, review what you have done, record any new tasks or procedures you have performed, and determine the extent to which you have met your objectives. Identify what you need to review and what skills you need to practice. Determine ways you can organize your time more effectively to increase your productivity.

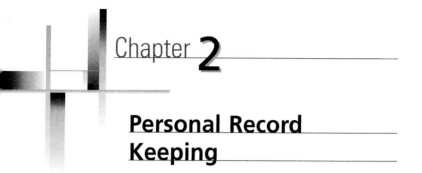

Chapter 2

Personal Record Keeping

This chapter contains forms to record information about the medical office, to identify daily objectives, to keep track of your schedule or hours worked, and to keep track of procedures you have performed. The list of procedures can also help you when you prepare your résumé. Take the time each day before and after work to record information so your personal records will be complete. Use these forms in the way that is most helpful to you. Their purpose is to help you get the most out of your experience.

TELEPHONE NUMBERS

Enter telephone numbers on the appropriate pages. Be sure to identify the telephone number and name of the contact person at your externship or office as well as your instructor (if you have one). Add telephone numbers (or telephone extensions) to this list when you are asked to make telephone calls, such as the answering service, laboratories, places where you schedule diagnostic tests, therapy departments, the hospital admissions department, and so on. Complete the page for emergency numbers including the number to activate emergency medical services, call an ambulance, the local poison control center, and so on.

PERSONAL NOTES

Use the Personal Notes section to record information about the medical office or clinic. This may include information such as the names of the primary care providers, the examination rooms used by each provider, personal preferences of various providers, laboratories used for different managed care plans, and other information you want to remember.

DAY PLAN AND MONTH PLAN

Use the day planning sheets to set goals and objectives for each day. Be sure to identify each day's date in the box provided. At the end of each day, you may want to check off those goals that were met, and you can write your new goals for the following day.

Use the monthly planning sheets to keep track of your schedule, hours worked, and any other information you want to record. Be sure to identify the month in the box at the top left.

LIST OF PROCEDURES PERFORMED

Keep a list of procedures you have performed at your externship. Enter in the appropriate date when you observed the procedure, when you performed it with supervision, and when you began to perform the procedure independently in the appropriate boxes. Your instructor or supervisor may want you to obtain the initials of the employee who has certified that you can perform the procedure independently, either in the box under the column labeled "Independent" or in the margin to the side of the box.

The procedure list is set up according to the list of entry-level competencies for medical assistants used by the Commission on Accreditation of Allied Health Education Programs. If you are in an externship, your instructor may want you to transfer this information to another form as part of your record keeping for the externship. When you create your résumé, use this list to identify procedures you can perform independently.

TELEPHONE NUMBERS

Medical Office:

Contact person:

Educational Institution:

Contact person:

TELEPHONE NUMBERS

TELEPHONE NUMBERS

EMERGENCY TELEPHONE NUMBERS

Emergency Medical System
(Ambulance, Fire, Police)

Poison Control Center

EMERGENCY NUMBERS

EMERGENCY TELEPHONE NUMBERS

PERSONAL NOTES

PERSONAL NOTES

PERSONAL NOTES

PERSONAL NOTES

☐ Mon ———————————————————————

————————————————————————————

————————————————————————————

☐ Tues ———————————————————————

————————————————————————————

————————————————————————————

☐ Wed ———————————————————————

————————————————————————————

————————————————————————————

☐ Thur ———————————————————————

————————————————————————————

————————————————————————————

☐ Fri ———————————————————————

————————————————————————————

————————————————————————————

Week of ———————————

← Clip for current week

☐ Mon ———————————————————————

———————————————————————————————

———————————————————————————————

☐ Tues ——————————————————————

———————————————————————————————

———————————————————————————————

☐ Wed ———————————————————————

———————————————————————————————

———————————————————————————————

☐ Thur ——————————————————————

———————————————————————————————

———————————————————————————————

☐ Fri ————————————————————————

———————————————————————————————

———————————————————————————————

Week of ———————————

DAY PLAN

Clip for current week ➝

☐ Mon _____

_____

_____

☐ Tues _____

_____

_____

☐ Wed _____

_____

_____

☐ Thur _____

_____

_____

☐ Fri _____

_____

_____

Week of _____

← Clip for current week

☐ Mon ————————————————————

————————————————————————————————

————————————————————————————————

☐ Tues ———————————————————

————————————————————————————————

————————————————————————————————

☐ Wed ————————————————————

————————————————————————————————

————————————————————————————————

☐ Thur ————————————————————

————————————————————————————————

————————————————————————————————

☐ Fri ————————————————————

————————————————————————————————

————————————————————————————————

Week of ———————————

DAY PLAN

Clip for current week ⟶

☐ Mon _____

_____

_____

☐ Tues _____

_____

_____

☐ Wed _____

_____

_____

☐ Thur _____

_____

_____

☐ Fri _____

_____

_____

Week of _____

← Clip for current week

☐ Mon ————————————————————

————————————————————————————

————————————————————————————

☐ Tues ———————————————————

————————————————————————————

————————————————————————————

☐ Wed ————————————————————

————————————————————————————

————————————————————————————

☐ Thur ———————————————————

————————————————————————————

————————————————————————————

☐ Fri ——————————————————————

————————————————————————————

————————————————————————————

Week of ——————————

DAY PLAN

Clip for current week ➞

MONDAY	TUESDAY	WEDNESDAY

← Clip for current month

THURSDAY	FRIDAY	SATURDAY/ SUNDAY

MONTH PLAN

Clip for current month →

MONDAY	TUESDAY	WEDNESDAY

← Clip for current month

THURSDAY	FRIDAY	SATURDAY/ SUNDAY

MONTH PLAN

Clip for current month ➞

MONDAY	TUESDAY	WEDNESDAY

← Clip for current month

THURSDAY	FRIDAY	SATURDAY/ SUNDAY

Clip for current month →

MONTH PLAN

OTHER NOTES

LIST OF PROCEDURES PERFORMED
ADMINISTRATIVE PROCEDURES

Perform Clerical Functions	Ob-served	Super-vised	Indepen-dent
Set up appointment matrix			
Make/Change appointments			
Schedule a diagnostic text			
Schedule a surgical procedure			
Complete a referral form			
Transcribe a dictated letter or report			
Prepare a medical record for a new patient			
Set up or use a tickler file			
File reports in a patient record			
File patient records			
Perform Bookeeping Procedures	Ob-served	Super-vised	Indepen-dent
Prepare charge slips for the day's patients			
Total charges on the charge slip			
Post charges to the patient ledger			
Record a patient's visit on a day sheet			
Balance a day sheet			
Prepare a bank deposit			
Reconcile a bank statement			
Write a check			
Create or examine an accounts aging record			
Write a collection letter			
Establish or maintain a petty cash fund			
Post adjustments			
Process credit balance			
Process refund			
Post NSF check			
Post collection agency payment			
Process Insurance Claims	Ob-served	Super-vised	Indepen-dent
Apply managed care policies and procedures			

	Ob-served	Super-vised	Indepen-dent
Validate insurance coverage for a procedure			
Obtain managed care referral or precertification			
Look up procedure codes			
Look up diagnosis codes			
Prepare insurance forms			
Send insurance information electronically			
Use a physician's fee schedule			
Other Administrative Procedures	Ob-served	Super-vised	Indepen-dent

CLINICAL PROCEDURES

Fundamental Principles	Ob-served	Super-vised	Indepen-dent
Use appropriate personal protective equipment			
Wash hands using medical asepsis			
Wash hands using surgical asepsis			
Dispose of hazardous waste correctly			
Sanitize or disinfect instruments			
Wrap instrument(s) for sterilization			
Operate the autoclave			
Specimen Collection	Ob-served	Super-vised	Indepen-dent
Perform venipuncture			
Perform capillary puncture			
Collect throat specimen			
Collect wound culture			
Instruct patient to collect random urine			
Instruct patient to collect clean-catch midstream urine			
Instruct patient to collect fecal specimen			
Obtain a sputum specimen			

Diagnostic Testing	Ob-served	Super-vised	Indepen-dent
Use methods of quality control			
Prepare specimen for transport to laboratory			
Test urine using reagent strip method			
Perform Clinitest			
Perform Acetest			
Perform Ictotest			
Prepare urine for microscopic examination			
Prepare a peripheral blood spear			
Test hemoglobin			
Perform microhematocrit			
Test blood for glucose or other chemicals			
Perform pregnancy test			
Perform rapd strep test			
Prepare a wet mount or hanging drop slide			
Prepare a dry smear for staining			
Innoculate culture plate			
Perform urine culture using a dip slide kit			
Screen and follow-up test results			
Take a 12-lead electrocardiogram			
Apply a Holter monitor			
Perform spirometry			
Patient Care	Ob-served	Super-vised	Indepen-dent
Screen patients on the telephone			
Manage emergency telephone calls			
Screen patients in the office			
Measure height			
Measure weight			
Take temperature using glass thermometer			
Take temperature using electronic/tympanic thermometer			
Measure pulse			
Measure respirations			

Measure blood pressure			
Measure head or chest circumference			
Record vital signs and measurements			
Obtain or review a patient's history			
Obtain a patient's chief complaint			
Prepare examination and treatment areas			
Check patients in			
Prepare patients for examination			
Assist with patient examination			
Measure distance visual acuity			
Test color vision			
Perform hearing testing			
Assist with flexible sigmoidoscopy			
Assist with a neurologic examination			
Assist with prenatal visit			
Assist with postpartum visit			
Put on sterile gloves			
Set up sterile field			
Prepare a patient for minor surgery			
Assist with minor surgery			
Apply or change a dressing or bandage			
Remove sutures or staples			
Perform an eye or ear irrigation			
Perform an eye or ear instillation			
Apply warm moist compresses			
Apply an ice pack			
Assist with cast application			
Administer oral or topical medication			
Administer an injection			
Take messages requesting medication refills			
Call medication refills to a pharmacy			
Document administration of medication			
Check contents of emergency box/crash cart			
Respond appropriately to emergency			

Other Clinical Procedures	Ob-served	Super-vised	Indepen-dent

TRANSDISCIPLINARY COMPETENCIES

Communication	Ob-served	Super-vised	Indepen-dent
Prepare a business letter			
Address an envelope			
Prepare outgoing mail			
Send a fax			
Respond to verbal communications			
Respond to non-verbal communication			
Answer incoming telephone calls			
Take a telephone message			
Get messages from an answering machine			
Place outgoing telephone calls			
Identify community resources			
Legal Concepts	Ob-served	Super-vised	Indepen-dent
Maintain patient confidentiality			
Perform within legal and ethical boundaries			
Maintain medical record as a legal document			
Document appropriately			
Perform risk management procedures			
Patient Instruction	Ob-served	Super-vised	Indepen-dent
Explain general office procedures			
Instruct individuals according to their needs			
Demonstrate the use of patient equipment			
Instruct patients to use ambulatory aids			

Teach self-examination (skin, breast, testes)			
Give follow-up instructions about medication			
Operational Functions	Ob-served	Super-vised	Indepen-dent
Take a supply inventory			
Stock a supply cabinet or exam room			
Prepare a purchase order			
Perform routine maintenance of equipment			
Use software to maintain computer systems			
Other Transdisciplinary Competencies	Ob-served	Super-vised	Indepen-dent

Administrative Procedures

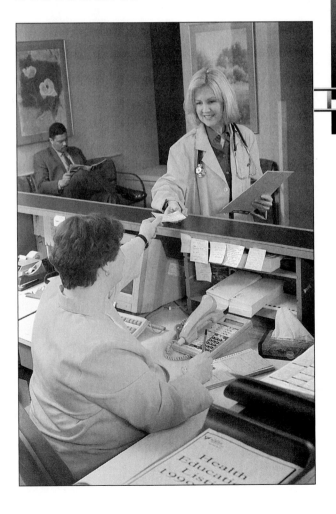

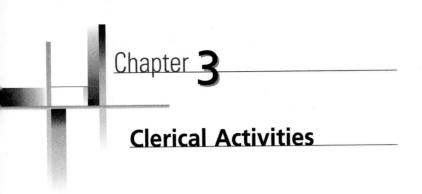

Chapter 3

Clerical Activities

TELEPHONES

The telephone may be your first point of contact with a patient or the community. Managing the telephone is one of the most important jobs in the medical office.

Incoming Telephone Calls

Incoming telephone calls can either be routed to the proper person electronically or through a person who answers the phone. During office hours, many offices use a human receptionist and turn on their electronic routing system for messages when the office is closed.

Find out if the office wishes you to pick up a ringing phone or if only the person assigned to answer the phone should answer. If you are asked to pick up, find out what greeting to use.

When you are asked to be responsible for incoming calls, make sure you have the right equipment and supplies:

- Message pad for taking individual messages
- Pen
- Telephone log to track incoming calls
- Scratch paper to write names and which line the caller is on when you are busy handling calls on many lines
- Directory for internal numbers to route calls properly
- Schedule, to see who is available to take any urgent calls
- Hands-free headset if you will be answering calls for a long time

Calls Referred to the Doctor

Some calls the medical assistant can handle. Other calls must be routed to a doctor or other licensed professional. If the doctor is with a patient, take a message (unless the caller is another doctor), and let the caller know approximately when the doctor will return the call. Calls that are referred to a doctor include:

- Providing a patient with test results
- Reports from patients of satisfactory or unsatisfactory progress
- Calls from other doctors
- Patients with medical questions
- Requests for medication or prescription refills

"Do-Nots" Regarding Incoming Calls

- Do not interrupt a doctor who is with a patient to take a call unless it is from another doctor.
- Do not put another doctor on hold except for the purpose of transferring the call.
- Do not discuss a telephone call with a doctor in front of a patient; speak to the doctor over the telephone rather than over the open intercom. You may also hand the doctor a message slip.

Handling Emergency Calls

If an emergency call comes in, follow office policy for handling emergency calls.

- Remain calm.
- Never put the caller on hold.
- If possible, get a doctor or other licensed professional to take the call immediately. (Write a note and have someone take it to the doctor, or have someone page the doctor on another line.)
- Get all pertinent information about the caller and the person experiencing the emergency (name, address from which call is coming).
- If you are alone, tell the person to go to a hospital emergency room.
- If the person does not have transportation or is too ill to drive, instruct him or her to call an ambulance (usually 911), or call the ambulance yourself if necessary.
- If you must call 911, do so using a different telephone if possible so that you do not have to put the emergency call on hold.
- If you have called 911, continue to speak to the individual until you hear the emergency response team arrive.

- If the emergency is a poisoning, refer the caller to the local poison control hot line, or call poison control yourself.

Problem Calls

Problem calls include calls from those who refuse to give information about the purpose of the call, calls with complaints, and calls from patients who have special problems. Each type of problem call must be handled in a different way:

If a caller refuses to give information about the purpose of the call:

- Listen carefully.
- Explain that you need a name, telephone number, and the purpose of the call so you can make sure the proper person responds to the caller.
- Instruct the caller to write a letter if he or she does not wish to leave the necessary information for a call back.

For a caller with a complaint:

- Listen carefully.
- Be patient.
- Tell the caller what you can do and what you will do.
- Refer the call to an appropriate person if possible.
- Understand that the caller is frustrated and the complaint is not personal.

If a caller has a special problem:

- Listen carefully.
- Get the caller's name and telephone number.
- If there is a language barrier, try to find a translator.
- If the caller seems confused, ask to speak with someone else who is there.
- If the caller is a child, ask to speak with an adult.

Outgoing Calls

- Never make personal outgoing calls, except in the case of a family emergency.
- Be sure you know the correct way of getting an outside line (e.g., dial 9, then the number).

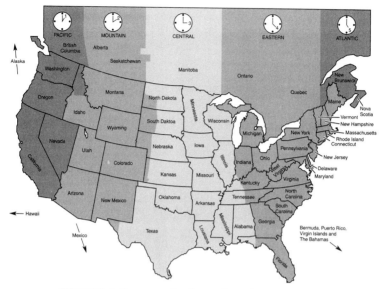

FIGURE 3–1. Time zones for the continental United States.

- **Don't use the incoming phone line to make outgoing telephone calls; patients will not be able to get through to the office.**
- If you place a long-distance call, be sure to verify that you are calling within normal business hours. Time zones for the United States are shown in Figure 3–1.

APPOINTMENTS

Appointment scheduling and appointment flow is a factor in patient satisfaction. Patients have little tolerance for waiting in a doctor's office. When learning to make appointments, it is helpful to observe someone making appointments for 1 or 2 hours before starting to make them yourself.

If you are asked to make appointments, either for patients in the office or over the phone, be sure to find out:

- How much time is allotted for different types of visits (new patient, established patients, follow-up visits, and so on)
- What information you need to take from a patient making an appointment

- Which type of appointment scheduling the office uses (appointment book or computer) and if the office double-books
- If appointments are booked centrally for all of the office's various sites

Daily Appointment Schedule

If you are checking patients in when they arrive, remember that the daily appointment schedule is the office's official, legal record of what patients were seen on a given day in a particular office. Any necessary changes (cancellations, no-shows, add-ins) should be made in red ink.

Sick and Urgent Visits

Sometimes doctors will see patients who need urgent appointments. There may be an emergency that occurs in the office. Other urgent care will be administered to patients who called that day and were given same-day, urgent appointments. Still others may even walk into the office without an appointment.

Find out if urgent visits are worked into the schedule of the patient's primary doctor or if one doctor is assigned to handle each day's urgent visits.

If patients call with urgent problems, refer to the office's procedure manual to determine what questions to ask in order to determine how serious the problem is and what type of appointment to offer.

SCHEDULING ADMISSIONS, DIAGNOSTIC TESTS, AND PROCEDURES

Many offices assist patients by scheduling all laboratory or diagnostic tests while the patient is still at the office, usually at the end of the visit.

When you begin working in a new office, create a list of all labs, radiology facilities, hospitals, or other diagnostic centers where the practice sends patients. Make sure to include a phone number and contact person for each facility.

When making an appointment for a patient's diagnostic test, be sure to have the following information available:

- Patient name and telephone number
- Type of test requested

- Required time frame for completion of the test
- Insurance information

Provide the patient with information about where the test will be administered and directions to the facility, the time the patient should arrive for the test, and any special instructions for test preparation.

Remember to document the information regarding the test in the patient's medical record.

CORRESPONDENCE

Medical offices generate a lot of correspondence, and preparing letters and envelopes may be a part of your job.

Sections of the Business Letter

The business letter has four sections:

- Heading (the sender's name and address); in most instances, doctors' offices use preprinted letterhead with the name of the practice, and each doctor's name
- Opening (date the letter is written; to whom the letter is being sent; and the greeting)
- Body (the substance of the letter)
- Closing (complementary close, signature, signature line, and any reference notations); if you are keying letters from dictation or from a doctor's notes, the doctor's initials should be capitalized, followed by a backslash, then your initials in lowercase

Figure 3–2 identifies the parts of a business letter.

Things to Find Out

If you are asked to prepare correspondence, find out:

- Where the office stationery supply is (letterhead and envelopes)
- What letter format to use (i.e., block, modified block, semi-block, or simplified)
- What complementary close to use (e.g., *sincerely, cordially,* or *with best regards*)

Ask the office manager or medical assistant who is working with you as a mentor for two or three old letters to use as examples to follow.

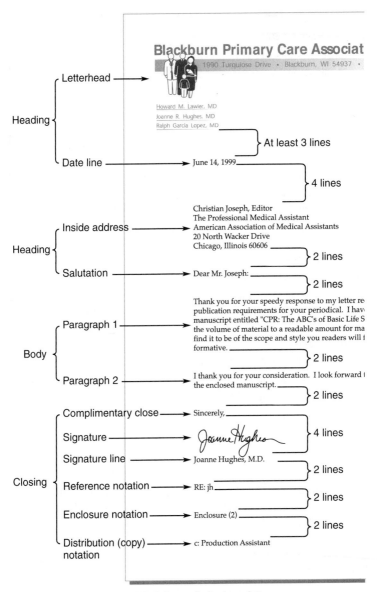

FIGURE 3–2. Parts of a business letter.

LETTER FORMATS

Block or Full Block Format—All lines are left-justified.

Modified Block Format—The salutation, complimentary close, and signature line begin at a tab stop in the center or to the right of the center. All other lines are left-justified.

Semi-Block Format—Same as modified block format, but paragraphs are indented five spaces.

Simplified Format—A subject line typed in all capital letters replaces the salutation and the complimentary close and signature lines are replaced by an all-capital-letter signature five lines below the letter's body.

The Envelope

The envelope should have the return address in the upper left-hand corner. The name and address of the person to whom the letter is being sent should be centered, using all capital letters and no punctuation (except for a hyphen between the first five numbers and the last four numbers of the zip code +4).

Any special instructions should be placed where they will not interfere with the postal service's optical scanning equipment. Figure 3–3 shows examples of properly prepared envelopes.

FILING

The patient medical record is a legal document that documents the care received or not received by a patient. As such, it must be maintained with care. In a large office that uses paper records, proper filing is of the utmost importance.

Filing Rules

Medical records are generally filed either alphabetically or by a numerical coding system. Guides are used to separate folders into sections, and outguides are used to indicate where a file has been removed.

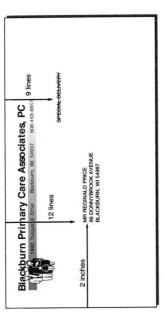

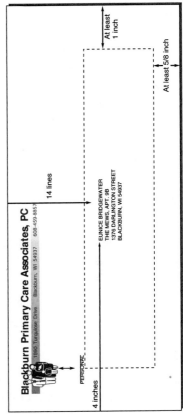

FIGURE 3–3. Properly formatted envelopes.

Alphabetic Filing

- Alphabetic filing uses legal names as the basis for determining where a file goes.
- The last name is the first filing unit (e.g., all *Smith* files are filed together, all *Walker* files are together).
- The first name becomes the second filing unit (e.g., *Alan Walker* is filed ahead of *Brittany Walker*).
- The middle name is the third filing unit. The record of a patient with no middle name is filed before the record of a patient with the same last and first names and also a middle name.
- Hyphenated last names are filed under the first of the two last names; if last names are not hyphenated, the final name is considered the last name.
- Abbreviations are filed as if spelled out. Prefixes such as *Mac-, Mc-, De, Van,* and so on are usually considered to be part of the last name for filing purposes. Find out exactly how they are treated in any particular office.

NUMERICAL FILING

- Each patient is given a unique identification number.
- Numerical filing preserves patient confidentiality.
- Numerical filing can be either consecutive or nonconsecutive (also called terminal digit filing).
- In terminal digit filing, the file number is broken up into groups (usually of two numbers) and filed by groups of numbers working from the final group back to the first group.

Locating a File

A patient record (in a file folder) has to be located when it is needed for an office visit or when the patient calls the office with a question. The file should be located according to the office guidelines for filing.

If you remove a patient file from its location, put an outguide into where the record file was removed. Return the file promptly after it has been used.

To locate a missing file:

- Look to see if any doctor or other employee has a stack of files that have not been replaced.

- If you are searching for a record and happen to find a different record that is misfiled, file it in its correct place immediately.
- If the office uses alphabetic filing by last name, look to see if the file was accidentally filed under the patient's first name.
- If the office uses colored labels, check the files for any record that stands out because the colored labels do not match those of the neighboring files.

Remember, when records are misfiled, the newest worker or the worker with the least experience is often blamed for the error by more experienced personnel. This may be you. You should not take it personally.

Chapter 4

Bookkeeping Procedures

Every medical office has its own bookkeeping systems and procedures. Most often today, bookkeeping is performed on a computer using a business accounting program. A medical office is a business; the service being provided is medical care.

During externship, you should ask to be shown how to use the office's bookkeeping system. This should always be done under supervision.

The patient account is made up of four parts:

- Charge slip (encounter form)
- Fee schedule
- Patient account ledger
- Day sheet

PREPARING CHARGE SLIPS BEFORE THE PATIENT VISIT

Working from the list of patients who will be seen that day, generate charge slips from the computer. The charge slips may be fed continuously through a printer with a tractor feed. If so, you must separate them carefully to avoid tearing them. Place each patient's charge slip with the medical record, using a paper clip to clip the slip to the front of the patient's folder.

If the office uses a pegboard system, prepare the day sheet and place the charge slips on the pegs "shingled" with the slip to be used first at the top.

Be sure to identify each patient carefully, using either the name, date of birth, or clinic number.

Charge slips may also be generated when the patient checks in, but in a busy office it is usually better to have all charge slips prepared ahead of time, even if a few patients cancel or do not show up for their appointments. If a patient is given an appointment for the same day, pull the patient's record and print a charge sheet.

BANKING PROCEDURES

Moving money into and out of the office's checking account involves three activities:

- Writing outgoing checks for payment
- Endorsing incoming checks
- Preparing a deposit slip

Writing Checks

Most offices use checks that come three to a page and have stubs on the side, on which the information on the check is written as a running record of payments and deposits. Information from the check should also be entered on the cash-disbursement record.

Some computer accounting programs allow you to generate checks from the computer and automatically post the check number and amount to the cash-disbursement record.

Checks are written on watermark paper, which makes them difficult to alter.

PROCEDURE FOR WRITING A CHECK MANUALLY

1. Assemble supplies.
2. Organize bills to be paid by opening envelopes and/or arranging invoices. Use a pen to prepare a check for each bill or invoice.
3. Write the name of the payee on the line of the check that says *Pay to the order of.*
4. Write the date on the line that says *Date.* If the check does not have a preprinted number, write the number of the check in the top right-hand corner, using the next unused number according to the check register.
5. Write the amount of the check in numbers next to the dollar sign and in words on the line below the name of the payee. Begin writing at the beginning of the line. When writing the

(continued)

PROCEDURE FOR WRITING A CHECK
MANUALLY *Continued*

numbers, use a decimal after the dollar amount and write the number of cents at a different level. (Example: $1,568.^{42}). When writing the words, remember that the word *and* is used only before the number of cents. Write the number of cents as a fraction over 100. Draw a line from the end of the fraction to the word dollars. (Example: One thousand five hundred sixty-eight and 42/100————dollars).

6. Write the invoice number, account number and/or purpose of the check on the line marked *For, Reference,* or *Memo.*

7. Record the date, check number, payee, amount of the check, and reason the check was written on the check stub in the checkbook or in the check register.

8. Record the information about the check on the cash-disbursement record as it was recorded on the check. If you are using a pegboard system, this step is unnecessary because a carbon on the back of the check automatically transfers the information to the cash-disbursement record.

9. Subtract the amount of each check from the balance in the check register and on the disbursement record as you write it.

10. If you make a mistake, draw a single line through the mistake, correct the error, and initial the correction.

11. If the check cannot be used, write the word *Void* across the check and enter the word *Void* in the check register. Place the voided check in the folder where accounts-payable records are kept.

12. Prepare an envelope in which to mail the payment or use a window envelope supplied by the vendor. Enclose the payment slip or a copy of the invoice. If using a window envelope, be sure that the payee's address is visible through the window.

13. If deposits were made to the checking account, enter the date and amount of the deposit and add the amount to the checking account balance in both the check register and on the cash-disbursement record.

14. Check all entries for accuracy. To proof entries, the total amount of each column of expenditures should equal the total amount of the column labeled *Amount.* The ending bank balance can also be proofed by adding the total of deposits to the beginning bank balance and subtracting the total amount of the checks written. This should equal the ending balance.

15. Place all invoices, bills, deposit slips, and voided checks in the accounts-payable folder.

Endorsing Checks

In order to cash a check or deposit it in a bank account, the check must be endorsed on the back. Most medical offices use a rubber stamp rather than handwriting an endorsement.

When endorsing checks, always use a restrictive endorsement (i.e., "For deposit only: [name of practice]"). Such an endorsement makes it nearly impossible for someone to forge a signature and cash a check meant for deposit. Checks are usually endorsed while preparing the bank deposit.

Bank Deposits

Deposits can be made in person at a bank teller window, by mail, or by a bank ATM (automatic teller machine) or night deposit box.

Every deposit must include the check(s) and/or cash being deposited, as well as a fully filled-out deposit slip.

PROCEDURE FOR PREPARING AND MAKING A BANK DEPOSIT

1. Obtain a practice deposit slip and place today's date on it.
2. Total all the cash and place the total on the line that says *Cash*.
3. Insert the amount of each check on the bank deposit detail with a reference number, which is usually the ABA number. This information may have already been recorded on the deposit section of the day sheet.
4. Total all the checks and place that total where it indicates for checks.
5. Total the cash and total amount of check for the total amount of the bank deposit. The total amount of this deposit should be equal to the amount in the payments column on the day sheet or accounts-receivable record for the given day.
6. Copy the deposit slip if a duplicate deposit record has not been made when creating the day sheet.
7. Place the deposit in a bank envelope or bank deposit bag and bring or send to bank.
8. A receipt should be given after deposit. Record the amount of the deposit on the accounts-payable record or record of disbursements.
9. File the bank deposit receipt and copy of the bank deposit detail in a labeled file folder.

On the deposit slip write the first part of the American Banking Association (ABA) number for the bank that the check is drawn on in the column labeled *Bank number* to identify the check and write the amount of the check in the column for payment by check.

COLLECTING COPAYMENTS AND COMPLETING CHARGE SLIPS

Copayment

Patients who are covered by managed care insurance programs must make a copayment at the time they visit the office. The copayment can either be taken before the patient is seen or at the end of the visit.

Enter the amount of the copayment on the charge slip when payment is made. Either give the patient a cash receipt for the copayment or give the patient a copy of the charge slip at the end of the visit to be used as a receipt.

Completing the Charge Slip

The doctor or other licensed practitioner places check marks on the charge slip next to the descriptions of all services provided. When the patient presents the charge slip at the billing desk (or when you take the folder from the doctor after the visit), use the fee schedule to enter the correct charges for each service.

If the patient has an insurance plan that includes a deductible, you need to see if the deductible has been met (this may mean looking in the patient ledger in the computer).

If a copayment has not been collected, collect it and deduct the copayment from the total, and the rest will be billed to the managed care company.

For Medicare patients and patients for whom you don't know how much insurance will pay, the patient may be asked to pay part of the bill, and any balance will be billed after insurance has paid.

ENTERING CHARGES IN THE PATIENT ACCOUNT

In a computerized billing system, each patient has a screen that shows the information about the patient's account. This includes charges, payments, adjustments, and the account balance. See Table 4–1 for definitions of common terms related to patient accounts.

When using a computer billing system, post a charge for each individual service provided that day. In most systems, this is done by entering the procedure code for each service. The office's fee schedule will have been entered previously, and the computer will automatically post the correct charge for each procedure code.

If a charge other than the regular charge is being entered, you can manually override the automatic posting.

Sometimes you will enter charges for each patient at the end of

TABLE 4–1	
Common Terminology for Entering Charges and Payments	
Account balance	The amount remaining in the account after all entries have been totaled
Accounts payable	Amounts the practice owes others
Accounts receivable	Amounts others owe the practice
Adjustment	Entry made to change an account, often to reflect a discount
Credit	The record of a payment received
Credit balance	A *negative* balance: the total of payments made is more than the total of charges
Day sheet	The daily record of financial transactions (daily journal in a pegboard system)
Debit	The record of a charge for a service
Disbursements	Money paid out
Invoice	A written statement describing a purchase or service and the amount due
Journal	The original record of financial transactions that identifies the accounts to which they belong
Ledger	A card or book to which records of financial transactions are transferred
Posting	Transferring information from one record to another
Proof	Validation of calculation
Received on account (ROA)	Designation used for payments that reduce the amount owed but are not payment in full
Trial balance	A method of checking the accuracy of calculations of accounts

individual visits. In other offices, you may be asked to enter all patient billing information at the end of the day.

Entering Payments and Adjustments

For a payment, made either by the patient or by an insurance company or the Medicare or Medicaid program, find the patient account ledger or computer account and post the payment.

Subtracting the payment from the balance gives you a new balance, which might be zero, positive (meaning the practice is still owed money), or negative (meaning the practice has been paid too much in total). A negative balance is called a credit balance.

When a payment is received from a managed care company or Medicaid, it will almost always be less than the full amount billed according to the office's fee schedule. After the payment is made, an adjustment should be made in the adjustment column so the account has a zero balance (or the amount of any unpaid patient copayment).

When a payment is made by Medicare, the balance is adjusted to the allowable charge as defined by Medicare plus any unpaid patient portion.

If a patient has a small credit balance, this is noted on a statement sent to the patient, and the patient can return the statement, requesting a refund. If a patient has a large credit balance, a refund check will usually be issued without the patient having to ask for it.

PETTY CASH

Petty cash is a small amount of cash (usually less than $100) kept for making small, nonroutine payments. These might include small donations made by the office (e.g., candy bars for the staff to snack on that are being sold by a patient to raise money for Girl Scouts, Little League, and so on).

Petty cash is kept separate from any cash used to make change for patients making cash payments.

Whenever petty cash is used, a receipt is made out for the payment, and the amount paid out is entered into the petty-cash journal.

To replenish the petty cash, a check is made out to *Petty cash* and cashed at the bank. The check number and amount are entered into the petty-cash journal.

PREPARING REPORTS

Most offices' computerized accounting systems can generate a number of different reports that can be used to analyze the practice's financial health. You need to find out which reports are routinely generated and how to produce them using the specific program used by the office. See Table 4–2 for a list of reports that can be created.

TABLE 4–2	
Reports for a Medical Practice	
Custom reports	Reports that can be generated according to a query or set of queries; this may include transaction journals to show each doctor's productivity.
Day sheet	A record of all transactions from a single day; in most programs, once the final day sheet for the specific period has been printed off, the program "closes" the day sheet so it cannot be altered; at this point, it may not be possible to print the information as a day sheet again
Insurance aging report	A breakdown of unpaid insurance claims, shown by how long the charge has been unpaid
Monthly or yearly summary	A summary of financial activity during each day of the current (or specified) period of time, either a month or the entire year
Patient aging report	A breakdown of unpaid patient charges, shown by how long the charge has been unpaid rather than by alphabetical order (e.g., all charges 60 days are shown together)
Practice analysis	This includes all the charges and payments for the practice for a defined period; it is usually generated monthly
Transaction journal	A record of transactions for a specific period; after a day sheet has been closed, you can usually print off the same information as a transaction journal by using the date of the day sheet

Chapter 5

Billing and Collections

Many medical offices today have billing specialists on staff who work on both patient billing and insurance billing. And most doctors request that patients pay what they must at the time service is provided.

However, there is often still a need to send patients bills, and smaller offices may continue to use one or more medical assistants to do the billing.

SENDING BILLS

Find out how billing is done in the office in which you work. Bills are sent out at regular intervals, known as the billing cycle. The most common cycle is weekly; the next most common is monthly.

Computer accounting programs can be used to generate bills, and many allow you to add written notations when bills are overdue, but some offices consider colored stickers that are added manually to be more effective than computer-printed notices.

COLLECTION ACTIVITIES

Bills are considered "overdue" if not paid within 30 days of the date the charges were billed (unless there is an outstanding credit agreement that sets the amount the patient will pay each month).

Overdue accounts are categorized as accounts over 60 days old, 90 days old, and 120 days old.

Collection activities begin with any bill that is over 60 days old. A computer-printed note or color-coded sticker should be attached to the bill stating that the account is overdue. The note should ask the patient to make a payment or to contact the office to make an arrangement for paying the bill over a period of time.

For bills that are over 90 days old, a sterner note should be attached and it may be helpful to place a telephone call at this point.

For bills that are over 120 days old, a "demand" letter should be issued, asking for payment in full.

Collection activities beyond notes and letters attached to bills include:

- Telephone calls to the patient to discuss the bill
- Turning the account over to a collection agency for collection
- Turning the account over to an attorney for collection
- Filing a lawsuit (usually in small-claims court)

If you call a patient to discuss paying the bill, be prepared to work out an arrangement for how frequently the patient will make payments and how much he or she will pay each time. If you make an agreement with a patient, you must write out a formal truth-in-lending agreement, even if no interest will be charged.

Remember, when calling patients about overdue bills:

- Do not call too early or late.
- Do not divulge to employers, neighbors, or other third parties that you are trying to collect on a bill from the patient.
- Do not threaten.
- Do not end the conversation on vague terms (always come to some sort of conclusion).
- Do not call repeatedly.

If you are asked to create individual collection letters instead of using computer-generated letters, remember:

- State clearly the amount of the outstanding balance.
- Show the date(s) that the charge(s) were incurred.
- Itemize the service(s) provided on each date.
- Show any amount paid by insurance.
- Describe any previous conversations and/or written agreements between the office and the patient about the bill.
- Clearly state the total balance due at this time, and identify a date (usually 10 days from the date of the letter) when the bill should be paid in full.

INSUFFICIENT-FUNDS CHECKS

If a patient's check is returned by his or her bank to your bank marked *insufficient funds* (also called *not sufficient funds* [NSF]), you should:

- Debit the patient's account for the amount of the check (you will have credited the account when the check arrived).
- Add a charge for the fee your bank has charged you for handling the insufficient-funds check, as well as for your time and effort (the office should have a standard charge for insufficient-funds checks).
- Call the patient and tell him or her that the check was returned and that you are adding the fees to the account.
- Encourage the patient to send a new check for the amount of the original bill and the fees.

TRACING SKIPS

A *skip* is an account for which there is insufficient information from which to pursue a collection. Some people "skip out" on debts deliberately, while others are simply forgetful about notifying every potential creditor about a change of address.

If you are unable to reach a patient at the address you have:

- Check to make sure there has not been a mistake made in the billing information (e.g., billing the wrong Smith).
- Send a bill by registered mail, with a return receipt requested (even if the period of time during which mail is forwarded has lapsed, the Postal Service will usually forward mail with special handling instructions).
- Try telephoning the individual at work (but never tell a third party that the reason you are calling is to collect on a bill).

ACCOUNTS THAT HAVE BEEN TURNED OVER TO A COLLECTION AGENCY

Collection agencies are in the business of collecting bills that have "aged out" of the collection cycle for small businesses. Collection agencies' behavior and techniques are highly regulated.

If you must find a collection agency to handle your office's bills:

- Get references from other businesses.
- Check any suggested agencies with the state Office of Consumer

Protection and/or Attorney General's Office to see if there have been complaints.

If a patient whose account has been turned over to a collection agency calls to discuss the bill, refer him or her to the collection agency. If a patient whose account has been turned over to a collection agency calls for an appointment, refer the call to the office manager or discuss the request with the doctor before making an appointment.

Any payments received from collection agencies must be posted to the day sheet on the day received, and posted to the patient's account. The difference between the billed amount and the amount collected (including the agency fee—usually 20%–40% of what is collected) is shown as a negative adjustment, and the practice's accountant will show it as a practice expense.

Chapter 6

Insurance Billing

Most insurance claim forms are generated in the medical office by computerized billing software. Some offices contract with a billing service and send information electronically from the office to the service, which then creates insurance claims (usually electronically) and bills for the office.

CODING

Computerized billing programs contain the most common procedures and diagnosis codes. Codes used for less frequently performed procedures or less frequently made diagnoses can either be added into the computer program or added individually to bills.

When looking up any medical codes for the purpose of billing, use the index to define the probable correct code, but **do not code from the index.** Always go to the narrative section and read the entire description of the code you have chosen as well as similar codes to determine which code is most appropriate. Improperly aggressive coding—that is, using the one of many similar codes that generates the highest reimbursement (often referred to as "upcoding")—is illegal.

CPT-4 Codes

- The CPT-4 manual provides narrative descriptions and five-digit codes for each procedure or service a doctor may perform for a patient.
- A two-digit "modifier" may be added to the code to indicate a more extensive procedure.
- Each section of the CPT-4 manual defines the procedures performed and services provided within a particular medical specialty

(e.g., evaluation and management, anesthesiology, surgery, radiology, pathology, or medicine).

- Codes for the service-oriented parts of medicine (evaluation and management) are differentiated by the completeness of the examination and the amount of skill required to manage the patient's condition.

HCPCS Coding

HCPCS (pronounced "hick-picks") coding is used by insurance companies that administer Medicare claims and has been adopted by many other insurance companies, which allows for billing using the HCFA-1500 form, sometimes known as a "superbill."

HCPCS coding uses three levels:

- Level 1 codes cover doctors' services and are the same as CPT-4 codes.
- Level 2 codes begin with a letter, A to V, and are consistent across the country.
- Level 3 codes begin with a letter, W to Z, and are inconsistent across the country.
- Level 2 and 3 codes cover categories of services covered by Medicare but not always covered by private health insurance (e.g., chiropractic, vision and hearing supplies, and transportation).

ICD-9-CM Coding

ICD-9-CM codes describe diagnoses. The purpose of ICD-9-CM codes is to track disease processes, classify causes of death, assist in medical research, and evaluate hospital-service utilization.

The ICD-9-CM manual has three volumes:

- Volume 1 is a tabular list of diseases, listed numerically by disease classification.
- Volume 2 is an alphabetic listing of diseases.
- Volume 3 contains both listings.

To find the proper ICD-9-CM code, use Volume 2, the index, to find the probable appropriate code. Cross-check this in Volume 1 to make sure it is most appropriate. For some diseases, Volume 1 contains a number of codes that show variations or nuances to the problem. Always code to the fourth digit, and code to the fifth digit if possible.

PREPARING THE INSURANCE CLAIM FORM

Most offices use the HCFA-1500 form as the standard insurance billing form (unless a patient's particular insurance company uses an individualized form). Office computerized billing systems generate the form.

PROCEDURE FOR COMPLETING THE INSURANCE CLAIM FORM

1. Enter information as required using capital letters and no punctuation.

2. Enter the name and address of the insurance company to whom the claim is being sent above the words *Health Insurance Claim Form*.

3. Complete the patient portion from information on the new patient registration form or from the patient's information form in the computer data base.

   Box 2:   Enter the patient's last name, first name, middle initial.

   Box 3:   Enter the patient's date of birth in the format MM DD YYYY, and the patient's gender (M or F).

   Box 5:   Enter the patient's address, using the two-letter state code; nine-digit zip code with a space between the fifth and sixth digits; telephone number with area code, space, three-digit prefix, space, then last four digits.

   Box 6:   Put an *X* in the box that defines the patient's relationship to the insured.

   Box 8:   Check the boxes that best describe the patient's marital and employment statuses. Determine if a college student is full time or part time.

   Box 10:   Check the correct box (*Yes* or *No*) to answer each question.

   Box 12:   If the office has on file the patient's signature on a similar form, enter *SOF* (for *signature on file*) in the box. If not, have the patient sign the form.

   Box 13:   If the doctor accepts assignment of benefits and the office has a signature on file, enter *SOF* in this box. If the doctor does not accept assignment of benefits, leave the box blank.

4. Complete the subscriber (insured) portion of the claim form using information in the patient data base.

   Box 1:   Place an *X* in the type of insurance being billed.

   Box 1A: Enter the identification number of the insured person.

PROCEDURE FOR COMPLETING THE INSURANCE CLAIM FORM *Continued*

Box 4: Enter the name of the insured person. If it is the patient, write *Same.*

Box 7: Enter the address of the insured person. If it is the patient, leave blank.

Box 9: If the patient is covered by a second insurance policy, enter the name of the insured, policy or group number (9a), insured's date of birth in MM DD YYYY form and gender (9b), employer's name (9c), and insurance plan or program name (9d). If the insured is not covered by a second policy, leave this blank.

Box 11: Enter information about the primary insurance, including the insured's group or FECA number, insured's date of birth in MM DD YYYY form and gender (11a), employer's name (11b), insurance plan or program name (11c), and if there is any other health benefit plan (11d). Many patients do not have a group insurance number.

5. Complete the physician or supplier information on the bottom half of the form.

Boxes 14 to 16 are not usually required for Medicare, Medicaid, Tricare, CHAMPVA, or most private insurance. If they must be filled in, use dates from the patient's medical record and/or the doctor.

Box 17: Enter the name of the doctor who referred the patient, if any.

Box 17a: Enter the identification number of the referring doctor.

Box 18: If the patient's claim is for a hospitalization, visit, or surgery performed when the patient was hospitalized, enter the dates of hospitalization. Otherwise leave blank.

Box 19: Leave blank unless instructed by the specific insurance carrier to use this box.

Box 20: Enter *No* unless billing Medicare for outside lab charges; for this, enter *Yes* and amount of charges.

Box 21: Enter the ICD-9-CM code(s) for up to four diagnoses.

Box 22: Leave blank unless the claim is a Medicaid resubmission; if Medicaid resubmission, enter code and original reference number.

Box 23: Leave blank unless you were given a preauthorization or precertification number by the patient's insurance company.

(continued)

PROCEDURE FOR COMPLETING THE INSURANCE CLAIM FORM *Continued*

Box 24A: Enter the date service began, in MM DD YYYY form, under *From*. If service occurred on only 1 day, leave *To* blank, otherwise enter when service ended.

Box 24B: Enter the code for the place of service. The code for a medical office is 11.

Box 24C: For medical service, leave this box blank. For other services (e.g., anesthesia) enter the correct code.

Box 24D: Enter the procedure code and modifier, if any.

Box 24E: Enter the number from Box 21 (1–4) of the diagnosis code that justifies the procedure.

Box 24F: Enter the charges, leaving a space between the number of dollars and cents, instead of using a period.

Box 24G: If charging for more than one of the same procedure (e.g., visits to a hospitalized patient on 3 consecutive days), enter the number of units of the procedure charged. Otherwise, enter *1*.

Box 24H: Leave blank unless the patient is enrolled in the Medicaid program for early, periodic, screening, diagnosis, and service (EPSDT).

Box 24I: Leave blank unless service took place in a hospital emergency room, in which case place an *X* in the box.

Box 24J: Leave blank unless there is coordination of benefits. If an individual doctor in a group practice has performed the service, place the first two digits of the doctor's NPI number in this box.

Box 24K: This box may be used for the last seven digits of a doctor's NPI number, as described earlier.

6. Enter information in Box 24, lines 1 to 6 for each procedure that is being billed to the insurance company. For more than six procedures, complete an additional HCFA-1500 form.

7. Complete the remaining boxes on the HCFA-1500 form.

Box 25: Enter the tax identification number for the practice. Indicate by checking the correct box if this is the social security number for an individual doctor or the employee identification number of a group practice.

Box 26: Enter the patient account number. Leave blank if there is no patient account number.

Box 27: Check *Yes* if the doctor accepts assignment of benefits or *No* if the doctor does not.

Box 28: Enter the total charges, with a space between the number of dollars and the number of cents.

PROCEDURE FOR COMPLETING THE INSURANCE CLAIM FORM *Continued*

Box 29: Enter the amount paid toward the current charges, including any copayment. If the amount is zero, leave the box blank.

Box 30: Enter the balance due, with a space between the number of dollars and the number of cents.

Box 31: Either have the doctor sign the form or use a stamp with the doctor's signature. Enter the date.

Box 32: Enter the name and address of the facility where the services were provided. If services were provided at the same address as the billing address, enter *Same*.

Box 33: Enter the name, address, and telephone number of the doctor, group, or supplier of services. Do not use punctuation. Leave a space between the city and the two-letter state code, and within the nine-digit zip code after the fifth digit. Leave spaces between the area code and digits 3 and 4 of the telephone number. Enter the NPI number for a group practice after *GRP*# or the PIN number for an individual doctor after *PIN*#.

8. Proofread the form and make corrections, then copy before mailing. Put the copy in the insurance-claims file, and mail the original.

PLACE OF SERVICE CODES COMMONLY USED FOR BILLING IN THE MEDICAL OFFICE

11 Office

12 Home

21 Inpatient hospitalization

22 Outpatient hospitalization

23 Emergency room—hospital

24 Ambulatory surgical center

25 Birthing center

26 Military hospital or clinic

31 Skilled nursing facility

32 Nursing facility

33 Custodial care facility

RESUBMISSION OF DENIED CLAIMS

If an insurance reimbursement claim is denied:

- Check the claim against the ledger and medical record to find any missing, incomplete, or incorrect information.
- Add all the information needed to justify the claim (i.e., copy of progress notes, or letter stating services performed).
- Enter resubmission on insurance submission log, and resubmit.
- Clip together copy of resubmission and copy of original submission.

COMMON ERRORS ON INSURANCE CLAIM FORMS

Avoid making the following errors when preparing insurance claim forms:

- Transposing (reversing the position of) the name of the patient and the name of the subscriber (guarantor)
- Transposing the primary and secondary insurance
- Transposing numbers in one of the identification numbers
- Missing signatures or the letters SOF
- Entering a diagnosis inconsistent with patient gender
- Using an incorrect diagnosis code or not coding to the fourth or fifth digit (ICD-9-CM)
- Using inaccurate procedure or service codes (CPT-4 or HCPCS)
- Missing modifier
- Not getting preapproval or preauthorization
- Using a diagnosis that does not justify procedures performed
- Total amount of billing does not agree with services provided
- Not providing physician SSN, EIN, or NPI number
- Not attaching required attachments (e.g., pathology report)
- Not completing boxes
- Place of service inconsistent with procedure code

Clinical Procedures

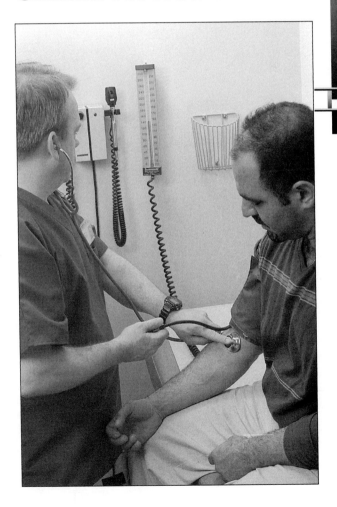

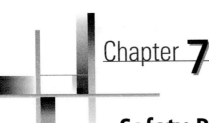

Chapter 7

Safety Precautions and Asepsis

The safety of office personnel and patients who visit the office is of paramount importance. A number of steps must be taken in order to ensure your safety, as well as the safety of your colleagues and patients. The safety precautions taken, including those for general asepsis, have three major goals:

1. To prevent the spread of infection
2. To prevent accident or injury
3. To prevent exposure to hazardous chemicals

PREVENTING THE SPREAD OF INFECTION

It is easier and cheaper to prevent infection than to treat infection after it has occurred. The five most often used methods of preventing the spread of infection-causing microorganisms are:

- Hand sanitizing
- Use of standard precautions and personal protective equipment (PPE)
- Disinfection and sterilization of instruments and surfaces
- Sterile technique
- Proper handling of specimens

Hand Sanitizing

There are two methods to sanitize the hands: hand washing and use of an alcohol-based hand rub. According to the Centers for Disease Control and Prevention (CDC) guidelines released in October 2002, hands must be washed using soap and water in the following situations:

- When hands are visibly soiled
- After using the restroom
- Before eating

The CDC guidelines recommend that hands that are not visibly soiled should be routinely decontaminated using an alcohol-based hand sanitizing rub, although it is also acceptable to wash the hands using antimicrobial soap. Situations where an alcohol-based hand rub should be used include:

- Before and after direct contact with patients
- After contact with intact skin
- After contact with a contaminated body site
- Before donning gloves and after removing them.

This recommendation was made because alcohol-based hand rubs significantly reduce the number of microorganisms on the skin, are fast-acting, and cause less skin irritation than washing with soap and water. They also take less time to use.

Use of Personal Protective Equipment

Items of PPE, such as gloves, masks, face shields or goggles, lab coat, and barrier gown or apron, are used to keep harmful microorganisms from coming into contact with the body.

Hand washing and appropriate use of PPE are part of what is known as *standard precautions,* which are taken to prevent any contact with body fluids that may transmit disease. The most commonly encountered body fluid is blood. In addition to standard precautions, there are also category-specific precautions as described in Table 7–1.

Standard precautions should be taken with every patient. Gloves should be changed after contact with a patient, and hands should be washed. Gloves should never be reused, should be removed by pulling from the cuff so that the contaminated surface ends up inside the glove, and should be discarded in a biohazard waste container (discussed later).

Disinfection and Sterilization

To kill microorganisms that are on a work surface or an instrument, disinfection methods such as soaking or boiling are used. After every use, equipment and instruments should be cleaned properly in order to remove visible residue, then rinsed and dried before disinfection or sterilization. This prevents the survival of microorganisms during the sterilization process. Wear gloves, an apron or lab coat, and face protection when sanitizing contaminated instruments.

TABLE 7–1
Precautions to Prevent Exposure to Pathogens

Precaution Type	Instructions
Standard precautions— used for all patients whenever there is a chance of exposure to blood or body fluids, including semen, vaginal secretions, cerebrospinal fluid, pleural fluid, peritoneal fluid, pericardial fluid, amniotic fluid, urine, feces, sputum, nasal secretions, breast milk, tears, and vomitus	1. Wear gloves to handle body fluids or for direct contact when a patient has open lesions of the skin or when touching the mucous membranes. 2. Wear a gown or lab coat or apron that is impermeable to fluid if there is any chance of splashes containing blood or body fluids. 3. Wear a mask and eye protection (such as safety glasses or goggles) if there is any chance of splashes to the face. A face shield may be substituted for the mask and glasses.
Category-specific isolation precautions—used in addition to standard precautions for patients with certain known diagnoses	
Airborne precautions—Used when patients have a known diagnosis of illnesses of transported airborne droplet nuclei	1. The patient should wear a mask in the waiting room. 2. Every health care worker who is not immune to the disease should wear a mask when providing direct care to the patient.
Droplet precautions—used when patients are known to have or are suspected of having illness transmitted by particle droplets	1. The patient should wear a mask in the waiting room. 2. Every health care worker should wear a mask when providing direct care to the patient.
Contact precautions—used for serious skin and wound infections caused by a variety of microorganisms	1. A health care worker who provides direct care to the patient should wear a disposable barrier gown with cuffs and gloves pulled over the cuffs. 2. If there is also a possibility of airborne or droplet transmission or splashes, a mask and eye protection should be worn. 3. Gowns and gloves should be removed before leaving the patient-treatment room. 4. The hazardous waste (including disposable gowns and gloves) should be double-bagged and disposed of promptly.

There are three levels of disinfection. The level of disinfection is determined by its ability to destroy the bacteria that cause tuberculosis, as well as bacterial spores.

- **Low-level disinfection** includes washing with disinfectant soaps and soaking in isopropyl alcohol. It is used to clean surfaces that have not been exposed to blood or body fluids.
- **Intermediate-level disinfection** kills bacteria and viruses, including *M. tuberculosis,* but does not kill bacterial spores. It is achieved by using a disinfectant solution to clean or soak the contaminated area or item. Commercial solutions are usually used for soaking instruments in the medical office, but to clean contaminated surfaces, 1:10 solution of household bleach (1 part bleach to 10 parts water) is often used. You should prepare fresh solution daily and allow any surface cleaned with this solution to air dry; drying time is an essential part of the disinfection process.
- **High-level disinfection** is obtained by using certain chemical solutions and soaking items to be disinfected in the solution for a longer period of time according to the directions on the label. High-level disinfection kills all microorganisms except high levels of bacterial spores. It is used for certain instruments that cannot be autoclaved without causing damage to instrument parts.

Sterilization is the killing of all microorganisms. Sterilization can be accomplished through the use of chemicals, gas, dry heat, or steam. Steam sterilization, using an autoclave, is most frequently used in medical offices.

Both wrapped and unwrapped items can be sterilized in an autoclave. Most medical instruments are wrapped for sterilization with paper wrap, cloth wrap, or sterilization pouches. Label the tape used to seal the package or sterilization pouch with the contents and date of sterilization.

The length of sterilization time depends on the:

- Temperature
- Pressure
- Number of items being sterilized
- Whether items are wrapped or unwrapped

Generally, items are placed in the autoclave at 250°F to 255°F at 15 pounds of pressure. Unwrapped items are sterilized for 15 minutes; wrapped instrument packages for 30 minutes; and large, double-

PROCEDURE FOR OPERATING AN AUTOCLAVE

1. Fill the reservoir tank to the correct level with distilled water.
2. Load the autoclave so there is room for steam to circulate.
3. Do not allow packages or items to touch one another.
4. Make sure containers are placed upside-down to prevent condensation inside the container.
5. Using the autoclave valve, allow water to flow into the sterilization chamber to the recommended level.
6. Close and tighten, or lock, the door to create a seal.
7. Turn on the autoclave, set timer and controls, and allow heat and pressure to rise to the recommended level.
8. When the correct temperature and pressure have been reached, set the timer for the amount of time necessary to sterilize the load.
9. When sterilization is complete, vent the autoclave.
10. Allow pressure to drop to zero, then "crack" the door (open door slightly to allow steam to escape). Keep hands and face away from opening to prevent burns.
11. Allow the items to remain in the autoclave until fully dry. If the autoclave has a drying cycle, set the timer so it will remind you when the drying cycle is over.
12. Remove items. Before storing them, check the sterilization indicators to be sure sterilization has occurred.

wrapped packages, for 45 minutes. Follow the manufacturer's directions for the particular model of autoclave that you are using.

Sterile Technique

While medical asepsis (also called clean technique) reduces the number of microorganisms present, surgical asepsis (called sterile technique) destroys all microorganisms.

Sterile technique is used whenever the doctor is going to penetrate below the skin or enter a sterile body cavity during a procedure. Sterile technique keeps harmful microorganisms and spores from entering the surgical incision or body cavity.

Sterile technique includes scrubbing the hands using the surgical aseptic hand-washing technique, wearing sterile gloves to touch sterile

instruments, and maintaining a proper sterile field during any procedure. See Chapter 13, Assisting with Surgery, for a discussion of aseptic
techniques.

Proper Handling of Specimens

All specimens of blood, body fluid, or tissue should be placed in a
spill-proof container to prevent any leakage during transport. Care
must be taken to deposit specimens inside the container and not
contaminate the container's outside in any way. In addition, specimens
are usually transported in a laboratory transport bag that protects
personnel handling the specimen and provides a pocket for the
laboratory requisition during transportation.

PREVENTING ACCIDENT OR INJURY

In order to prevent accidents or injuries from occurring in the office, it
is necessary to keep floors dry (or mark recently cleaned wet spots with
safety markers) and to keep materials in storage containers and out of
hallways and doorways. Instruments should be kept stored until ready
for use. Electrical equipment should be plugged into wall sockets. Fire
extinguishers should be present in the laboratory and any room with
oxygen, and the staff should be trained in their use. An emergency-exit
plan should be drawn up and practiced regularly.

PREVENTING EXPOSURE TO HAZARDOUS CHEMICALS

Any doctor's office that performs laboratory testing on specimens (even
the most simple tests) has hazardous chemicals in the lab. The best way
to prevent exposure to hazardous chemicals is to follow laboratory
rules for safety, including:

- Washing hands when entering and leaving the lab
- Following standard precautions at all times, including the use of
  appropriate PPE
- Not touching face, mouth, or eyes with hands, pens, or laboratory
  equipment
- Never using a mouth pipette to draw specimens
- Labeling and storing chemicals properly

  All potentially hazardous chemicals must be inventoried. A manual

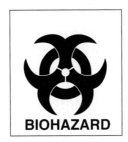

FIGURE 7–1. The biohazard logo is used to identify specimens of blood or body fluids and hazardous waste.

must be created that contains a material safety data sheet (MSDS) for every hazardous chemical found in the office. Find out where the manual is, and be sure to refer to it if you are exposed to a chemical or if a spill occurs. If you order a new product for the office, request an MSDS from the vendor or manufacturer.

Even when using protective eye wear, there is a possibility that hazardous or caustic chemicals will get into your eyes. For this reason, each laboratory has an eyewash station. If you get chemicals in your eyes, flush them thoroughly at the eyewash station for at least 5 minutes.

A lab that uses hazardous chemicals should also have a shower area for employees who become exposed to chemicals to thoroughly clean themselves before they leave the lab. This is not only for their own safety but also so they don't contaminate other people in the office.

Disposal of Hazardous Waste

Every medical office produces hazardous waste. Biohazard waste bags and rigid biohazard containers are marked with the universal biohazard sign, shown in Figure 7–1.

Plastic biohazard bags are used to dispose of soiled gloves, gauze squares, bandage and dressing material, exam-table paper, and other "soft items."

Rigid biohazard containers are used to dispose of "sharps," such as hypodermic needles and syringes, scalpels, suture needles, broken glass lab equipment, and lancets used for finger sticks.

Cleaning staff does not handle hazardous waste. If you are asked to prepare hazardous waste containers for removal by an outside contractor:

- Wear gloves, mask, and protective eye wear.
- Close each bag securely.
- Double-bag—put the bag inside another hazardous waste bag—if there is any chance of leakage.
- Place bags in the secure place where the contractor picks them up.

Reusable linens that have been soiled with biohazardous materials—cloth lab coats, cloth gowns and drapes, and so on—must be either laundered in the office or packed in special leak-proof bags and removed by a laundry able to handle contaminated material.

Handling Spills

Spill cleanup kits must be available to deal with spills of hazardous chemicals or biohazardous fluids. You need to know where the kits are kept and how to use them.

If a spill occurs involving either hazardous or caustic chemicals or biohazardous material:

- Notify the office's designated safety officer immediately.
- If the safety officer designates you to clean up the spill, get a spill kit.
- Put on a barrier gown with knitted cuffs, gloves, mask, and eye protection.
- Follow the directions on the spill kit to clean up the bulk of the spilled material.
- Disinfect the area where the spill occurred.

If the spill involves mercury, do not clean it up yourself. Call the local HazMat agency—authorities from the state's environmental protection agency who deal with hazardous material spills—to clean the spill. Keep staff and patients away from the area where the spill occurred.

Chapter 8

Interview and Documentation

INTERVIEWING THE PATIENT

When interviewing a patient, you need to make sure you are obtaining all of the necessary information and presenting that information in a format that is useful to the doctor. To do this, make sure you are familiar with the patient history and other forms used by the office you work in and with the various ways individual doctors like a patient history and statement of the chief complaint presented.

Although the patient has been asked questions about his or her billing and insurance at the front desk and often has filled out a written health history questionnaire while waiting to be seen, you should take the patient to a private area to discuss his or her medical history and the current health problem that has brought the patient to the office that day.

In addition to providing confidentiality for the discussion, a private place also helps to avoid distraction and allows the patient to stay focused on the interview. This is very important in completing the patient interview within the allotted time and getting the patient ready for the examination.

You must manage the interview and not allow the patient to. At the same time, you must be empathetic and attentive to the nuances of what the patient is saying.

OBTAINING THE MEDICAL HISTORY

Working with the office's medical history form, either ask the patient each question in order to complete the form or ask the patient to fill out the form and go over it to be sure all information is complete. If the patient completes the form, he or she usually does this in the waiting room before being placed in an exam room.

You should be familiar with the correct pronunciation of each term on the form and be able to explain what information is needed from the patient.

OBTAINING THE CHIEF COMPLAINT

The chief complaint is the reason the patient has come to the office today.

Ask, "What brings you to the office today?" or "What is the reason for your visit today?"

Ask the patient to describe the symptoms—changes in physical condition that the patient experiences through his or her senses or as a sensation, such as pain, nausea, or itching; or as a feeling, such as anger or sadness. Symptoms are subjective complaints, meaning they are experienced in different ways by different people.

Also note any signs—changes that can be observed and/or measured—such as redness, swelling, or pallor. Signs are objective, meaning they can be observed by others and characterized in a consistent way by many observers.

A discussion of the chief complaint is sometimes known as the *history of the present illness* (HPI). You should try to obtain seven pieces of information that can be used to completely describe the patient's chief complaint:

- Location
- Quality
- Severity
- Chronology
- How it began
- What makes it better or worse
- Associated symptoms

Location

Location gets at where exactly in the body the symptom is felt. Ask, "Where exactly does it hurt?" or "Can you show me exactly where it hurts?" to get the patient to pinpoint the location.

Quality

The quality of a symptom refers to how one describes or characterizes the symptom. The quality of pain can be described as sharp, throbbing, dull, burning, crampy, and so on. Ask the patient to use an analogy if he or she can't describe the pain (e.g., "It feels like someone is sitting on my chest" is the way one might describe a heart attack).

Severity

The severity helps describe quantitative aspects of an illness. Are symptoms intense, moderate, or mild? You might ask the patient to rate the symptoms on a scale of 1 to 10, with 1 being undetectable and 10 being extremely uncomfortable.

Chronology

Chronology asks the patient to explain how the illness began and how the symptoms have changed over that time. Some medical history forms have subsections for this, called onset, duration, frequency, and change over time.

How It Began

How it began is self-explanatory, but it may be important to determine what the patient was doing when the symptoms began, to see if a particular activity, or a particular place, could have had an effect on the onset of the illness or episode (e.g., chest pain with vigorous activity, asthma attack at the zoo).

What Makes It Better or Worse

Ask what the patient has done to try to alleviate the symptoms and if there has been any effect. Certain symptoms are often relieved by exercising, sitting or lying in a particular position, bowel movement or urination, or other changes. Include any medications the patient has taken and if they have helped. Look up the names of medications, if necessary, to be sure you spell them correctly.

Associated Symptoms

Associated symptoms gets at the "minor" symptoms that occur around any disease process (e.g., a sore throat or ear pain is often accompanied by a fever and/or stuffy nose; stuffy nose with no fever hints that the sore throat is being caused by a virus, while fever with a sore throat but no stuffy nose suggests a bacterial infection; rash may be caused by allergies, but it may also be caused by something as simple as a change in medication or even laundry detergent).

DOCUMENTATION

Documentation of the patient history and statement of the chief complaint is extremely important. The chief complaint should be documented with the length of time the patient has had the symptoms, accurately and precisely.

Use medical terminology and appropriate abbreviations, as shown in Figure 8–1.

Remember, everything in a patient's medical record is a legal document. If you document directly into the medical record, follow the guidelines given later. If you record vital signs and the chief complaint on a sticky note for the doctor to incorporate into his or her dictation, be sure to label the note with the patient's name.

If you use the patient's own words, make sure to put them in quotes. Make sure to state only your observations and the objective data you have obtained from various tests. Do not put your subjective feelings or determinations into your documentation. Do not use a term that is a medical diagnosis. See Figure 8–2 (p. 85) for sample documentation of the chief complaint.

Many doctors use the SOAP format for documentation, and you may be asked to write your findings using this format. The SOAP charting format has four main components:

1. <u>S</u>ubjective impressions
2. <u>O</u>bjective data
3. <u>A</u>ssessment
4. <u>P</u>lan

Subjective Impressions

These are impressions the patient has about his or her own condition, the things the patient describes that only the patient can experience— the symptoms.

Parts of the history and physical examination

H & P	history and physical examination
PE	physical examination
CC	chief complaint
HPI	history of present illness
FH	family history
SH	social history
OH	occupational history
ROS	review of systems

General

c̄	with	>	greater than
dc, D/C	discontinue	<	less than
DOB	date of birth	Δ	change
Dx	diagnosis	↑	increase
Hx, H/O	history of	↓	decrease
ETOH	alcohol intake	°	degree
NKA	no known allergies	Ø	without
pt	patient	@	at
Rx, Tx	treatment	♂	male
s̄	without	♀	female
SP, S/P	status post (has had in the past)	×	times (used with a time measurement, as in 2 weeks)
stat	immediately		

FIGURE 8-1. Abbreviations used to document the history and chief complaint.

Figure continued on following page

Body locations		Signs and symptoms	
lt or Ⓛ	left	S & S	signs and symptoms
rt or Ⓡ	right	c/o	complains of
LA	left arm	BM	bowel movement
RA	right arm	LMP	last menstrual period
LL	left leg	mod	moderate
RL	right leg	N & V	nausea and vomiting
abd	abdomen	sl	slight
LLQ	left lower quadrant of the abdomen	SOB	shortness of breath
LUQ	left upper quadrant of the abdomen		
RLQ	right lower quadrant of the abdomen		
RUQ	right upper quadrant of the abdomen		

FIGURE 8–1 Continued.

Patient Interview #1

Medical Assistant: *What is the reason for your visit today?*
Patient: *My throat has been sore since Tuesday.*
Medical Assistant: *That's three days now isn't it? Have you had any fever?*
Patient: *I don't know. I don't think so.*

Sample charting

6/12/99	c/o sore throat x 3 days.............................S. Williams, CMA

Patient Interview #2

Medical Assistant: *Why have you come to see the doctor today?*
Patient: *I have had terrible stomach pain all morning*
Medical Assistant: *can you show me where it hurts?*
Patient points to area 3 inches below belly button in the middle.
Medical Assistant: *Have you taken anything to relieve the pain?*
Patient: *I took Maalox but it didn't help?*
Medical Assistant: *When did you take it?*
Patient: *At 9:30 this morning.*

Sample charting

6/12/99	Pt. c/o severe midline abdominal pain since this a.m. Took
	Maalox this a.m. s̄ relief.............................S. Williams, CMA

Patient Interview #3

Medical Assistant: *What is the reason for your visit today?*
Patient: *I have been having really bad headaches.*
Medical Assistant: *When did the headaches begin?*
Patient: *Well, I always have headaches occasionally, but lately
I've had two or three a week, like for the last two weeks.*
Medical Assistant: *Are they in the front or back, can you show me?*
Patient: *They are all over. It feels like someone is hammering my head.*
Medical Assistant: *What do you do when you have one?*
Patient: *I have to lie down. I've been taking ibuprofen, but it doesn't help.*

Sample charting

6/12/99	Pt. c/o severe generalized headaches for two weeks, 2-3 per
	week. Says "it feels like someone is hammering my head."
	Has taken ibuprofen without relief................................
	....S. Williams, CMA

FIGURE 8–2. Sample interviews and appropriate documentation.

Objective Data

This is the information that can be observed or measured—the signs. Objective data include measurements and vital signs.

Assessment

This is a summary of what the subjective and objective information, taken together, means. In a doctor's charting, it is often written as a first impression of a possible diagnosis. A medical assistant should always avoid using any term that is a medical diagnosis.

Plan

This is a written description of the diagnostic tests the patient will undergo, medications that will be prescribed, treatments that will be given, and follow-up the patient will receive.

OTHER GUIDELINES FOR DOCUMENTATION

- If you do chart directly in the patient record, double-check to make sure it is the correct record.
- Use only blue or black ink when writing in a patient chart.
- All entries to a patient record are added in chronologic order.
- Draw a line through any unused lines to avoid charting out of chronologic order.
- If you make a mistake, do not erase. Draw a single line through the mistake and initial it. If you make a correction on a different date than the original entry, date and initial the correction.

Chapter 9

Assisting with Examinations and Treatments

As a medical assistant, you will be asked to take on various responsibilities during examinations and treatments, depending on the procedures followed by the office in which you work and the specific preferences of each doctor.

In most offices, you will be asked to take vital signs and assist patients into various positions during the exam. You may also be asked to set up instruments for procedures, treatments, and diagnostic tests and to take care of the exam room and instruments before and after an exam or treatment.

VITAL SIGNS AND MEASUREMENTS

The medical assistant usually takes vital signs and measurements at every office visit. Follow the office procedure for taking and documenting vital signs.

Height and Weight

The medical assistant usually measures height or length of infants and children at every well-baby or well-child visit. The head and chest circumferences of infants are also measured and recorded. For adults, the height is measured at the initial visit, and weight is usually measured at every visit.

Temperature

In some offices, the medical assistant takes a patient's temperature at every visit, but in others he or she takes a patient's temperature only when there is a possible infection or signs and symptoms of a fever.

When taking temperature, use the method appropriate for the patient's age and health status.

Table 9–1 is a comparison of the various methods for taking temperature. Figure 9–1 (p. 90) shows Fahrenheit/Centigrade temperature conversions.

Pulse

Pulse should be recorded for adults and children.

If the patient's pulse is regular, measure for 30 seconds and double; if the pulse is irregular, measure for a full 60 seconds.

Document the pulse rate and include the volume only if the pulse is extremely strong (bounding) or weak (thready). Document whether the pulse is irregular.

The pulse is usually taken apically for an infant. Note the rate at 30 seconds in case the infant becomes too restless for you to measure the pulse for a full minute.

Respirations

Respirations should be recorded for adults and children.

If the patient's respirations are regular, measure for 30 seconds and double; if the respirations are irregular, measure for a full 60 seconds.

Count while the patient is unaware—keep your hand on the wrist so that the patient thinks you are still measuring pulse. This discourages the patient from talking or altering his or her respiratory rate.

Table 9–2 (p. 91) shows the normal range for heartbeat and respirations at various ages.

Blood Pressure

Blood pressure is the pressure of the blood against the walls of arteries. The systolic pressure refers to the pressure when the heart's ventricle contracts. The diastolic pressure refers to the pressure when the ventricles relax between heartbeats.

When measuring blood pressure:

- Select the proper cuff size; the width of the cuff should be one-third larger than the diameter of the arm.
- Apply the cuff snugly with the center of bladder over the brachial artery.
- Pump up to 30 mm Hg above the expected blood pressure.

TABLE 9–1
Comparison of Methods for Taking Temperature

Method	Time Needed	Normal Temperature	Special Considerations	Accuracy
Axillary	10 minutes	≈ 97.6°F; may be as much as 2.2°F below core temperature	Assist patient to hold arm tightly against side.	Least accurate
Oral—glass mercury	3–5 minutes	≈ 98.6°F; may be as much as 0.8°F below core temperature	Do not use for children under 5; not suitable for mouth breathers, patients on oxygen, inaccurate after recent eating, smoking, chewing gum, drinking.	Good
Oral—electronic	10–60 seconds	≈ 98.6°F; may be as much as 0.8°F below core temperature	May be used safely for children who can hold probe under tongue; other considerations same as oral glass mercury thermometer above.	Good
Oral—disposable	60 seconds to 3 minutes	≈ 98.6°F may be as much as 0.8°F below core temperature	May be used for children who can hold probe under tongue; other considerations same as oral glass mercury thermometer above.	Fairly good
Tympanic—electronic	2 seconds	≈ 98.6°F	May be inaccurate if tip does not point to eardrum or if patient has excessive wax in the ear.	Good
Rectal—glass mercury	3–5 minutes	≈ 99.6°F; may be as much as 1°F above core temperature	Patient must lie still to avoid breaking bulb or stem of the thermometer or perforation of rectum.	Most accurate
Rectal—electronic	10–60 seconds	≈ 99.6°F may be as much as 1°F above core temperature	Patient must lie still to avoid perforation of the rectum.	Most accurate

Data from web article by Robert Knies at Emergency Nursing World [online]. Available: http://enw.org/Research-Thermometry.htm [February 13, 2000].

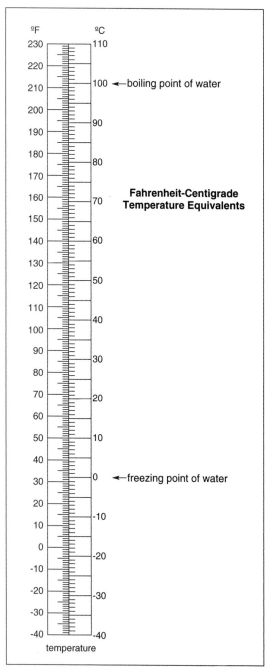

FIGURE 9–1. Fahrenheit-Centigrade temperature equivalents.

TABLE 9–2 Normal Range of Heartbeat and Respirations at Various Ages		
Age	**Normal Range of Pulse Rate**	**Normal Range of Respiratory Rate**
Infants	70–170	30–60
Children (1–7 years)	80–120	18–30
Older children (7–12 years)	60–110	20–26
Adult	60–100	14–20

- To determine how high to pump, for a current patient, check the chart for the blood pressure on the last visit.
- To determine how high to pump for a new patient, palpate the systolic pressure. To do this, place your first finger on the radial pulse and pump up cuff. Note where the pulse disappears (approximate systolic pressure). Add 30 mm Hg to that point when auscultating the blood pressure.
- Release valve so blood pressure indicator decreases 2 to 4 mm Hg per second.
- Note when the first sound is heard (systolic pressure).
- Note when the last sound is heard (diastolic pressure).
- Deflate the cuff fully.
- Record the blood pressure as a fraction (e.g., 122/82) using only even numbers. Note which arm blood pressure was taken on. Note whether the patient was lying down or standing.
- If you had trouble getting a reading (e.g., if the patient spoke, someone came into the room, or there was another distraction) allow the arm to rest for at least a minute before pumping the cuff again.

Measuring Height of Fundus

The fundus is at the base of the uterus. During pregnancy, the height of the fundus is measured during every exam. Fundal height should correspond to the assumed gestational age of the fetus.

To measure the height of the fundus, measure from the tip of the symphysis pubis to the top of the fundus.

Fundal height larger than expected for the assumed gestational age

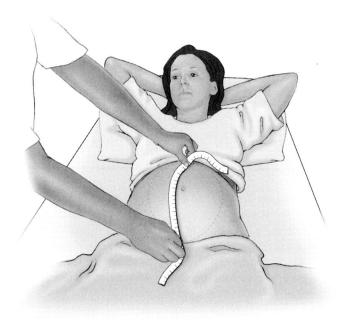

FIGURE 9–2. Measuring the height of the fundus at a prenatal visit.

(determined by calculating from the date of last menses) may signify multiple fetuses.

Fundal height smaller than expected usually signifies poor fetal development.

Figure 9–2 shows measurement of fundal height.

POSITIONS USED FOR EXAMINATIONS AND TREATMENTS

When preparing a patient for an examination, be sure to know the doctor's preference for how the patient should be dressed and positioned for the beginning of the exam. Usually, the patient should be sitting at the end of the examination table.

Positions that the patient may be asked to get into during the course of an examination include:

- Sitting
- Supine
- Semi-Fowler's

- Dorsal recumbent
- Left-lateral (Sims')
- Lithotomy
- Prone
- Knee-chest
- Trendelenburg
- Standing

In the photos that accompany the position descriptions, transparent draping is used to illustrate the position the patient should be in under the drape. In an office, opaque paper or cloth draping will be used.

Sitting

As shown in Figure 9–3 (p. 94), the patient sits at the end of the table with a drape over his or her knees. This position is used for examination of head, eyes, ears, nose, and throat (HEENT), chest, and reflexes.

Supine

As shown in Figure 9–4 (p. 94), the patient lies on his or her back, with a drape covering the lower abdomen. This position is used for examination of the abdomen, breasts, and reflexes.

Semi-Fowler's

As shown in Figure 9–5 (p. 95), in semi-Fowler's position, the patient is on his or her back with the head of the exam table raised 45° so the patient is in a semi-sitting position, with a drape covering the legs and abdomen. The legs should be supported with the exam-table extension. This position is used for patients with problems that make it difficult to breathe in the supine position.

Dorsal Recumbent

As shown in Figure 9–6 (p. 95), in the dorsal recumbent position, the patient lies on his or her back with knees bent, with a drape covering the legs and abdomen. This position is used for examination of the genitalia and rectum.

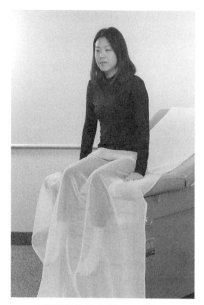

FIGURE 9–3. Sitting position.

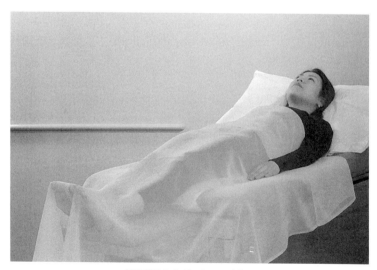

FIGURE 9–4. Supine position.

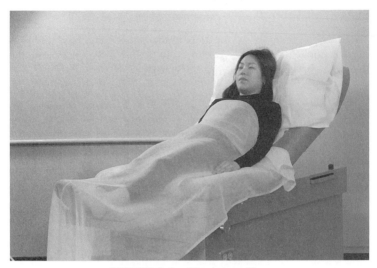

FIGURE 9–5. Semi-Fowler's position.

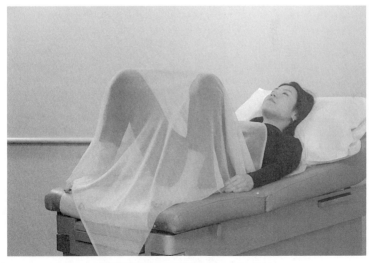

FIGURE 9–6. Dorsal recumbent position.

Sims' (Left-Lateral)

As shown in Figure 9–7, the patient in the Sims' position lies on his or her left side with the knees bent up to 90°, with a drape covering the lower body. This position is used for examination of the rectum and lower back.

Lithotomy

As shown in Figure 9–8, in the lithotomy position, the patient lies on her back with feet in stirrups, with a drape over the legs and lower abdomen. This position is used for examination of the female genitalia and pelvis.

Prone

As shown in Figure 9–9, in the prone position, the patient lies on his or her abdomen with legs extended, with a drape covering the lower body. This position is used for examination of the back and the back of the legs.

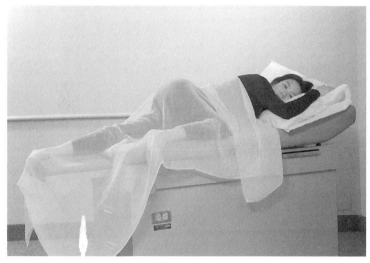

FIGURE 9–7. Sims' (left-lateral) position.

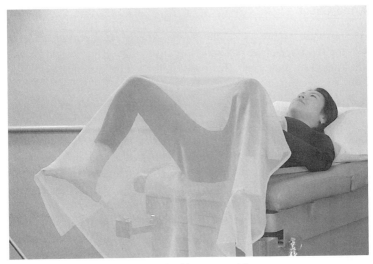

FIGURE 9–8. Lithotomy position.

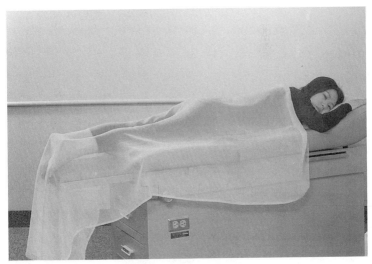

FIGURE 9–9. Prone position.

Knee-Chest

As shown in Figure 9–10, the patient kneels on the exam table to assume the knee-chest position, supporting his or her weight on the chest, elbows, and arms. This position is used for examination of the anus and rectum.

Trendelenburg

In Trendelenburg position, the patient lies on his or her back, with the head lower than the body. A patient is placed in this position when there are signs of hypotension (low blood pressure) or shock, to increase blood flow to the brain. In an emergency room, the cart on which the patient is examined can usually be adjusted to lower the head. In the physician's office, if this position is required, it may be necessary to improvise. Have the person lie backward on the examination table, with the legs over the backrest, as shown in Figure 9–11.

Standing

The standing position is used to examine balance. Male patients stand facing the doctor for the doctor to perform testicular and hernial exams,

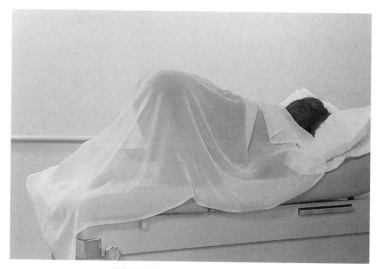

FIGURE 9–10. Knee-chest position.

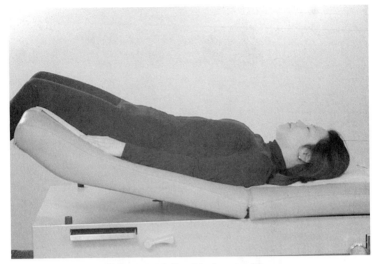

FIGURE 9–11. Trendelenburg position.

and facing the exam table, often bent over, for the doctor to perform a rectal exam.

Position for Lumbar Puncture

As shown in Figure 9–12, the patient is placed in a position for a lumbar puncture to widen the spaces in the lumbar spine, presenting the doctor with the largest possible space to insert the needle to remove cerebrospinal fluid. The medical assistant usually must hold the patient in this position during the procedure to prevent a sudden movement.

INSTRUMENTS USED IN EXAMINATIONS

Table 9–3 lists the instruments used in a physical examination and the portion of the examination they are used for.

CARE OF EXAMINATION AREA AND INSTRUMENTS

Before the first use of an examination room each day, and between examinations, the room must be prepared for each new patient.

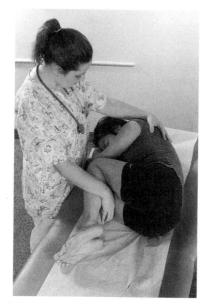

FIGURE 9–12. Position for a lumbar puncture.

Equipment and surfaces such as countertops and/or chairs might need to be sanitized, disinfected, and/or sterilized.

Preparation of the exam room includes:

- Stocking and placing in position all necessary equipment and supplies
- Replacing the examination table paper if necessary (table paper lasts about 75 patients per roll)
- Cleaning the room, discarding used supplies in wastebasket or appropriate biohazard container
- Sanitizing and disinfecting surfaces and instruments if necessary

When preparing for the patient examination:

- The stethoscope ear pieces and bell should be cleaned with alcohol wipes.
- Used instruments should be stored in soaking solution until they can be cleaned.
- Contaminated surfaces should be disinfected with a 1:10 bleach solution (wear heavy rubber gloves).
- Glass thermometers need to be cleaned. Wearing gloves, wash with

soap and cool water, then rinse with cool water. After drying, place in disinfectant such as Cidex for 30 minutes to 1 hour. Rinse in cold water, dry, and store.

To sanitize other instruments:

- Wear heavy-duty rubber gloves, apron or lab coat, and eye protection.
- Collect all soiled instruments and rinse in cold water, then place gently in a basin of warm, sudsy water.
- One instrument at a time, use a scrub brush to scrub all surfaces, rinse thoroughly under hot water, and place on paper towels to dry. (Leave instruments with ratchets and cutting faces open.)
- With more paper towels, dry instruments gently.
- Clean and rinse basin thoroughly, clean rubber gloves, store gloves with basin.
- Wash hands.

TABLE 9-3
Instruments Used for the Physical Examination

Patient Position	Part Examined	Instrument(s)
Sitting	Head and neck	Stethoscope
	Eyes	Ophthalmoscope, penlight
	Ears	Otoscope with disposable ear speculum, tuning fork
	Nose	Penlight, nasal speculum, substances to smell
	Mouth	Glove, tongue blade, penlight
	Chest	Stethoscope
	Arm reflexes	Percussion hammer
Supine	Abdomen	Stethoscope, tape measure
	Leg reflexes	Percussion hammer
	Sensation	Safety pin, tubes of hot and cold water
Standing	Hernia (male)	Glove
	Prostate (male)	Glove and lubricant
	Rectum (male)	Glove and lubricant
Lithotomy	Pelvis (female)	Gloves, vaginal speculum, slide or Thin Prep solution, cervical brush, cervical spatula, fixative
	Rectum (female)	Glove and lubricant

EMERGENCY CARE

An emergency can occur at any time, so you must be prepared to deal with any kind of emergency situation.

- Know where emergency phone numbers are (there should be an emergency number list by every telephone extension).
- Know where emergency supplies and equipment are.
- Know where fire extinguishes are located, and know the emergency evacuation plan for both your office itself and the building.

Emergency Supplies and Equipment

The emergency box/crash cart should be checked regularly to make sure all equipment is present and that no supplies or medications are past their expiration dates. The accompanying boxes list all of the equipment and supplies that should be present in an emergency box/crash cart, as well as how to check them. Table 9–4 describes medications commonly used in an emergency.

FIRST AID SUPPLIES

1. Adhesive tape
2. Hot and cold packs
3. Slings, triangle bandage, tourniquets
4. Sterile and nonsterile dressings in various sizes
5. Alcohol wipes
6. Bandages, gauze, bandage scissors
7. Tongue blades
8. Personal protective equipment such as gloves, goggles, masks
9. Splints
10. Elastic bandages and gauze bandages
11. Stethoscope
12. Penlight

ADDITIONAL SUPPLIES USUALLY FOUND ON A CRASH CART

1. Airways in various sizes
2. Manual resuscitator (Ambu-bag)
3. Endotracheal tubes (ETTs) in various sizes
4. Laryngoscope
5. Oxygen, and supplies for administering it
6. Syringes and needles in various sizes
7. Medications in cartridges, with holders for the cartridges
8. Sphygmomanometer
9. IV equipment, including bags, tubing, tourniquets, boards, pole, butterfly needles, and/or intracaths to start an IV
10. A defibrillator and/or cardiac monitor (usually kept on top of the crash cart)
11. Suction catheters and suction equipment (usually)

TABLE 9–4
Medications That Should Be in Every
Emergency Box/Crash Cart

Medication	Description
Epinephrine (adrenaline)	A vasoconstrictor, used to improve circulation; also for use in coronary conditions, or as a bronchodilator to relieve respiratory distress; crash carts often contain preloaded syringes for intracardiac administration
Atropine	May be used to decrease body secretions while increasing respiratory and heart rates; also a smooth muscle relaxant, it relieves hypermotility of the intestinal tract and gastrointestinal cramps
Digoxin (Lanoxin)	A cardiotonic with a fairly rapid action if given parenterally; used for congestive heart failure
Lidocaine (Xylocaine)	0.5% or 1.0% solution used as a local anesthetic; lidocaine in various strengths is also given intravenously or intramuscularly to prevent or treat cardiac arrhythmias; crash carts often contain preloaded syringes for use in cardiac arrest

(continued)

TABLE 9–4
Medications That Should Be in Every
Emergency Box/Crash Cart *Continued*

Medication	*Description*
Syrup of ipecac	An emetic. Used in cases of poisoning
Apomorphine HCl	A rapid-acting emetic
Isoproterenol (Isuprel, Medihaler-Iso, and other brands)	An antispasmodic for bronchospasm; also a cardiac stimulant; should be kept in both injectable and inhalable forms
Diphenhydramine hydrochloride (Benadryl)	An antihistamine used to relieve the effects of histamines, or for mild to severe allergic reactions
Metaraminol (Aramine)	Used to raise blood pressure for a patient in shock
Amobarbital sodium (Amytal) or phenobarbital	Sedatives for anxiety or anticonvulsants, used to relieve seizures
Diazepam (Valium)	A sedative and anticonvulsant; it is also an effective muscle relaxant when given intravenously
Activated charcoal	Binds with some poisons to prevent absorption
Furosemide (Lasix)	Diuretic used to treat congestive heart failure
Methylprednisolone or prednisone	Corticosteroids used for allergic reactions and for respiratory symptoms
Nitroglycerin tablets	Vasodilator used to treat angina pectoris
Phenytoin (Dilantin)	Anticonvulsant used to treat seizures
Glucagon, orange juice, glucose paste, sugar packets, dextrose 50%	Used to treat hypoglycemia
Insulin	Used to reduce elevated blood sugar
Sodium bicarbonate, injectable	Stored in preloaded syringes to restore acid/base balance during cardiac arrest
IV dextrose in saline or water, as well as lactated Ringer's solution	Used for intravenous hydration

PROCEDURE TO CHECK THE EMERGENCY BOX/ CRASH CART

1. Obtain the inventory control sheet for the emergency box/crash cart.
2. Open box or cart and check each drawer or compartment.
3. Identify presence of each item on the inventory control sheet.
4. Note on the sheet which items are missing. Then recheck each item for its expiration date.
5. Remove any items that have passed their expiration date. Note on the sheet which items were removed.
6. Discard any items beyond expiration appropriately.
7. Using the inventory sheet, obtain items that were missing or discarded and restock the box or cart.
8. Note that items missing or expired were restocked. Date and initial the inventory sheet.

IF YOU HAVE TO CALL AN AMBULANCE, BE PREPARED WITH THE FOLLOWING INFORMATION

1. Exact location of the victim(s)
   - Street name and house number
   - Floor and room number (if applicable)
2. Number of victims involved
3. Condition of the victim(s)
   - Complaints
   - Symptoms
   - Progression of symptoms
4. Name of caller, relationship to the victim(s)
5. Care that has already been given

Common Emergencies

The most common emergencies you might encounter in the medical office are:

- Allergic and anaphylactic reactions
- Severe bleeding
- Diabetic emergency
- Angina and heart attack
- Burns

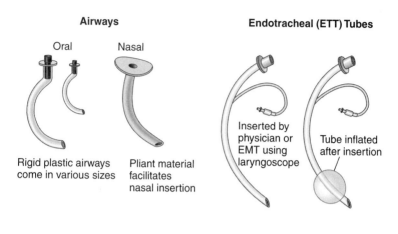

Airways   **Endotracheal (ETT) Tubes**

Oral   Nasal

Rigid plastic airways   Pliant material   Inserted by   Tube inflated
come in various sizes   facilitates   physician or   after insertion
                         nasal insertion   EMT using
                                                  laryngoscope

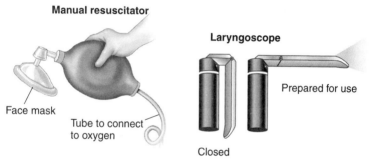

Manual resuscitator

                                          Laryngoscope

                                                            Prepared for use

Face mask
                Tube to connect
                to oxygen   Closed

FIGURE 9–13. Emergency equipment to establish or maintain an airway.

At some point, you may need to perform cardiopulmonary resuscitation (CPR). You need to remember to recertify in CPR when necessary. Many medical offices bring in a trainer to recertify the entire staff at once, or pay for your certification classes.

When dealing with an unconscious patient, check the *ABCs* (i.e., the three most important things to check):

- **Airway.** When unconscious, a person's tongue may relax and obstruct the airway. The tongue must be cleared from the airway to allow for passage of air to the lungs.
- **Breathing.** Look, feel, and listen for breathing. Look for a rising and falling of the chest. Feel for a pulse. Listen for air moving through the nose and mouth. Figure 9–13 illustrates equipment used to establish or maintain an airway and assist with breathing.

- <u>C</u>irculation. Make sure you can feel the patient's pulses in the neck, wrist, and foot.

Allergic and Anaphylactic Reactions

An anaphylactic reaction occurs when a normally inoffensive foreign body stimulates an atypical immune-system response. An allergic response can include itching, sneezing, watery eyes, a feeling of itching or tightness in the throat, and/or the presence of raised patches of skin called hives.

Anaphylaxis is an acute and life-threatening allergic reaction that can occur within minutes of exposure to a substance one is allergic to (called an allergen).

Physiological changes that occur during anaphylaxis can be fatal. Massive amounts of histamine are released, which causes bronchospasm, vasodilation, and a dramatic drop in blood pressure.

Constant monitoring of vital signs is necessary for a patient having an anaphylactic reaction. If necessary, the doctor may administer or order epinephrine to be injected subcutaneously, and the site may be massaged vigorously to enhance absorption.

Anaphylaxis may be a reaction to a medication, an insect bite or sting, or food (e.g., shellfish allergy). Before administering any medication, look in the patient's medical record and check with the patient (and/or the patient's parent or caregiver) about any medication allergy.

If an anaphylactic reaction occurs, obtain help from the doctor or primary care provider as soon as you notice that the patient is experiencing distress. Prepare to draw up and administer epinephrine if it is ordered. Also obtain supplies to administer oxygen if ordered by the physician.

Controlling Severe Bleeding

Symptoms of excessive external bleeding are obvious blood seepage through any covering over a wound; restlessness; cold, clammy skin; thirst; rapid and thready pulse; rapid and shallow respirations; a drop in blood pressure; and a decrease in the level of consciousness.

The best way to control severe external bleeding is to apply pressure directly to the site. Pressure usually controls capillary or venous bleeding. If direct pressure does not control the bleeding, it is necessary to find a pressure point where an artery lies close to the skin so the blood flow to a wider area can be slowed, giving the bleeding site a chance to clot. The pressure points are illustrated in Figure 9–14.

A pressure bandage should be used. A tourniquet should not be used in an office situation, in which transportation to a hospital is available; a tourniquet should be used only in a remote area where loss of blood flow and possible tissue death is preferred to a patient bleeding to death.

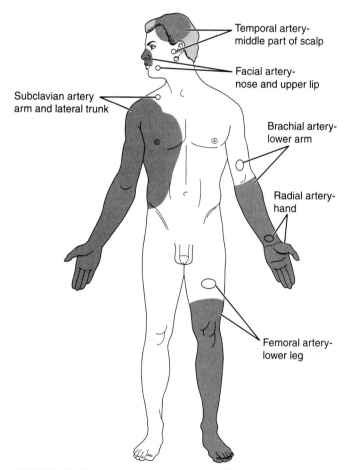

Temporal artery-
middle part of scalp

Facial artery-
nose and upper lip

Subclavian artery
arm and lateral trunk

Brachial artery-
lower arm

Radial artery-
hand

Femoral artery-
lower leg

FIGURE 9–14. Pressure points and areas where bleeding can be reduced.

Diabetic Emergency

A patient with diabetes may incur one of two different emergency situations. One is hyperglycemia (high blood sugar), sometimes called diabetic coma. The other is hypoglycemia (low blood sugar), often called insulin reaction.

Hyperglycemia has a gradual onset, usually taking place over a 12- to 18-hour period. Hyperglycemia is treated with insulin to help the body metabolize the blood sugar.

Hypoglycemia has a rapid onset, often occurring in a matter of minutes or an hour. Hypoglycemia is treated with rapid intake of sugar or glucose. A conscious individual is given fruit juice, candy, or soft drinks. An unconscious individual is given IV fluids.

Because hypoglycemia occurs more rapidly than hyperglycemia and can cause permanent brain damage if not treated promptly, the first response to an unconscious diabetic or a diabetic who is conscious but incoherent should be to give sugar and observe the response. If the problem is actually hyperglycemia, insulin can be given later.

COMPARISON OF DIABETIC COMA AND INSULIN REACTION

	Diabetic Coma	*Insulin Reaction*
Cause of the condition	Lack of insulin	Too much insulin
Onset	Gradual	Rapid
Skin	Warm, dry	Cool, clammy
Breath	Fruity or acetone odor	Unremarkable
Respirations	Deep	Shallow
Pulse	Rapid, thready	Rapid, bounding
Thirst	Intense	Not marked
Hunger	May or may not be present	Intense
Vomiting	Common	Rare
Abdominal pain	Common	Rare
Blood glucose level	Hyperglycemia: > 200 mg/dL	Hypoglycemia: < 60 mg/dL
Urine glucose	Present	Absent

Angina and Heart Attack

Angina is a clinical syndrome that accompanies arteriosclerotic cardio-vascular disease. Chest pain is caused by narrowing of the arteries, which in turn cause arteriospasm.

Angina attacks usually last 15 to 30 minutes. Rest may reduce the pain. To treat an angina attack, have the patient get into a semi-reclined position. Nitroglycerin can be given sublingually as a vasodilator to relieve symptoms and repeated after 5 minutes. If two nitroglycerin tablets do not quell the pain, the patient should be transported to a hospital emergency room.

You should know where nitroglycerin is stored in the office and be sure it is replaced every few months to be sure it stays potent. The patient also sometimes carries his or her own supply. If a patient complains of chest pain, do not attempt to have the patient lie flat. Place the patient in semi-Fowler's position to reduce the oxygen demand on the heart and obtain help as soon as possible. Be prepared to take an electrocardiogram and/or administer oxygen if ordered.

A heart attack (also called a myocardial infarction) occurs when blood flow to the heart is severely reduced or completely cut off, usually because of blockage of a major vein leading to the heart. Symptoms of a heart attack in men is left-chest pain that often radiates down the left arm or into the left side of the neck and jaw, the throat, or the left shoulder. It is often accompanied by nausea and vomiting, shortness of breath, and profuse sweating. Many women do not experience these symptoms but may have a feeling of severe heartburn, indigestion, or other gastrointestinal symptoms.

An ambulance is usually called as soon as a patient is suspected of having a heart attack so that he or she can be transported immediately to the emergency room.

Burns

Burns can be caused by thermal, chemical, or electrical accident. Burns are generally classified by the amount of the body surface involved and the penetration of skin layers.

To treat first-degree burns (the least severe), use cool-water dressing or immersion in cool water, pat dry, and apply a sterile dressing.

For second-degree burns, which usually blister, immerse in cool water, pat dry, apply antiseptic ointment if ordered, and apply a sterile dressing. Remove any jewelry from the burned area because swelling will occur.

To treat third-degree burns (sometimes called *full-thickness burns*), cover the burns with a sterile dressing and treat the patient for shock. Do not try to remove clothing. Transport the patient to an emergency room immediately.

Figure 9–15 illustrates the three types of burns.

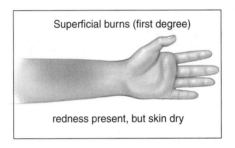

Superficial burns (first degree)

redness present, but skin dry

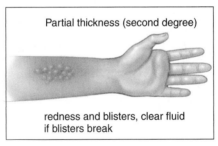

Partial thickness (second degree)

redness and blisters, clear fluid
if blisters break

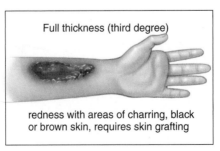

Full thickness (third degree)

redness with areas of charring, black
or brown skin, requires skin grafting

FIGURE 9–15. Different types of burns.

ESTIMATING BURN SEVERITY

Minor burns are third-degree burns that cover less than 2% of body surface, or second-degree burns that cover less than 15% of an adult's body surface, or less than 10% of a child's body surface.

Moderate burns are third-degree burns that cover between 2% and 10% of body surface, or second-degree burns that cover from 15% to 25% of an adult's body surface, or from 10% to 20% of a child's body surface.

Major burns are third-degree burns that cover more than 10% of body surface area, or second-degree burns that cover over 25% of an adult's body surface, or over 20% of a child's body surface.

Burns to the hands, feet, or genitalia are always considered major burns. Burns to individuals who are high risk or have associated fractures are always considered major burns. Electrical burns are always considered major burns.

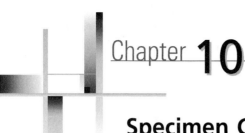

Chapter **10**

Specimen Collection

As a medical assistant, you will either collect specimens (e.g., blood, throat, and wound specimens for culture) or instruct patients how to collect the specimens themselves (e.g., urine or feces).

You may be responsible for testing these specimens in the office laboratory, or you may be responsible for properly labeling, storing, and/or transporting these specimens to an outside lab for testing.

Proper collection of specimens is imperative. Improperly collected specimens can yield poor or inconclusive results. When collecting specimens:

- Always use standard precautions.
- Know how various specimens should be stored (e.g., refrigeration or chemical additives).
- Know how to package a specimen in a biohazard transport bag.
- Find out how to fill out a laboratory requisition form for the particular lab your office uses to perform outside testing.

VENIPUNCTURE

Venipuncture for collection of venous blood for testing is usually carried out using a vein on the inside of the elbow. See Figure 10–1 (p. 114) for the names and locations of the veins of the forearm.

The blood may be collected in evacuated tubes or in a syringe. If a syringe is used, the blood is transferred to evacuated tubes, which often contain additives. See Table 10–1 (p. 115) for a list of evacuated tubes with a description of their additives.

The puncture may be made using a double-pointed needle, a standard needle, or a butterfly needle. Figure 10–2 (p. 116) shows the

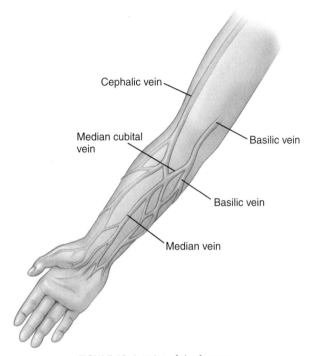

FIGURE 10–1. Veins of the forearm.

GUIDELINES FOR OBTAINING BLOOD SPECIMENS

1. Have appropriate types and sizes of tubes (for every 1 mL of serum needed, draw 2.5 mL of whole blood).
2. Wash hands and change gloves between each procedure.
3. Properly identify the patient.
4. Review the test requisition.
5. Assemble all the necessary equipment before beginning the draw. Be sure to have extra tubes available in case a tube has no vacuum.
6. Use an alternative cleaning method for the draw site, rather than an alcohol pad, if a blood alcohol level is to be drawn. Hydrogen peroxide or soap and water may be used.
7. To avoid damaging blood cells, don't use a needle with a gauge smaller than 23.

TABLE 10–1
Evacuated Tubes Arranged in Order of Draw for Evacuated-Tube Method of Venipuncture

Stopper Colors*	Additives	Testing Purpose	Handling Instructions
Yellow	Additive: Sodium poly-anetholesulfonate (SPS)	Blood and body fluid cultures	Ensure sterility upon collection
Plain red	None	Serum testing, immunology, serology, blood bank, chemistry	Allow to clot at least 40 min, centrifuge; access to clot for blood bank testing
Light blue	Sodium citrate (anticoagulant)	Coagulation testing utilizing plasma	Centrifuge immediately upon collection or separate plasma and refrigerate and test w/in 4 h or freeze
Green	Sodium/lithium heparin (anticoagulant)	Plasma; used for chemistry plasma testing or when patient is on anticoagulant therapy	Centrifuge immediately and separate to analyze
Lavender/ purple	Ethylenediamine-tetra-acetic acid (EDTA) (anticoagulant)	Whole blood; hematology testing and manual erythrocyte sedimentation rate (ESR); malarial stains	Mix well; analyze within 4 to 8 h of collection
Red-and-black marble; ("tiger top")†	No additives but contains a gel serum separator	Serum; most chemistry analysis; ideal for most chemistry instrumentation	Allow to clot at least 40 min; centrifuge and analyze; no access to clot
Gray	Potassium oxalate/sodium fluoride (anticoagulant)	Plasma; glucose determinations, esp. when delay in testing anticipated; alcohol levels	Centrifuge and separate to analyze

*Stopper colors are based on Becton-Dickinson tubes.
†The manufacturer recommends treating this tube as one containing additives and using it in the order listed above, but some labs consider it a tube without additives and use it immediately after a plain red-stoppered tube.

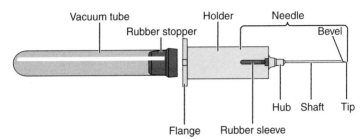

FIGURE 10–2. Components of the evacuated-tube method for venipuncture.

parts of the evacuated-tube system, which is most commonly used because several tubes of blood can be collected at the same time.

If a patient has small veins, veins that collapse, or veins that roll, you may prefer to use either the syringe method or the butterfly-needle method to obtain a specimen.

When collecting blood using the butterfly needle, after preparing equipment, greeting and explaining the procedure to the patient, donning gloves, and assessing the patient's veins:

- Pick up prepared holder or syringe with butterfly needle and tubing attached, and remove needle cover from butterfly needle.
- Hold the blue wings in dominant hand with needle at 15° angle, stabilize vein, and puncture vein with one quick motion.
- Allow the needle to rest in the vein supported by the wings. Rotate if necessary until the needle rests flat.

If using evacuated tubes, push the first tube onto the needle and allow it to fill by vacuum action. If using a syringe, slowly pull back on the plunger until the syringe has filled with the desired amount of blood.

If you drew blood into a syringe, transfer it to evacuated tubes as described previously.

If You Have Problems Finding the Vein

If you do not obtain blood after making the puncture, gently palpate over the needle to determine if the tip of the needle is above the vein, is beside the vein, or has penetrated through the vein. Based on your assessment, make one or two attempts to enter the vein in order to

PROCEDURE FOR VENIPUNCTURE USING THE EVACUATED-TUBE METHOD

1. Wash hands.
2. Prepare supplies and equipment per the lab slip or encounter form, including gathering all of the appropriate tubes for the tests ordered (color coded in correct order of draw), screwing the posterior needle into the holder securely and opening an alcohol pad.
3. Identify the patient, explain the procedure, and confirm the requisition and any special preparations (e.g., fasting). Arrange collection tubes in the proper order of draw.
4. Assess veins on both arms, using a tourniquet. If this takes longer than 1 minute, remove the tourniquet, allow the arm to rest, and reapply before proceeding.
5. Put on gloves, cleanse site with alcohol, and dry with a gauze square.
6. Pick up the holder in your dominant hand and place the first tube in the holder without pushing it onto the needle.
7. Remove needle cover.
8. Stabilize and penetrate the vein in one quick motion.
9. Allow holder to rest on your fingers, push the tube on to the needle, and allow it to fill from the vacuum in the tube.
10. Withdraw the tube when full and change tubes as necessary, with the holder remaining in place.
11. When last tube begins filling, release tourniquet.
12. Remove last tube from holder, remove needle from arm, and place gauze square over puncture to stop bleeding. Tell the patient to hold the gauze firmly over the puncture site and to keep the arm straight.
13. Dispose of needle in a rigid biohazard container, gently rotate any tubes with additives, label tubes or place preprinted barcoded labels on tubes.
14. When the bleeding has stopped, put a bandage on the puncture site and discard the gauze squares and gloves in the biohazard container.
15. Wash hands; document.

avoid having to start again, but do not "dig around" excessively because this can cause a hematoma. If the needle is too shallow, advance it slightly. If it is too deep, pull back slowly. If it is beside the vein, pull back slightly and then advance at an angle to penetrate the vein. If any part of the needle bevel comes above the skin, the vacuum in the tube will be lost, and you will need to change to a new tube in order for blood to flow. See Figure 10–3 for a summary of problems that can prevent blood from entering the evacuated tube or syringe.

PROCEDURE FOR VENIPUNCTURE USING THE SYRINGE METHOD

1. Prepare equipment, greet and identify the patient, explain the procedure, assess the patient's veins, put on gloves, and prepare the site as described in the procedure for venipuncture using the evacuated-tube method.

2. Prepare the evacuated tube(s) to hold the blood in a test-tube rack in the correct order of draw (tube[s] with additives first, tube[s] without additives last).

3. Remove the needle cover from syringe.

4. Holding syringe in dominant hand at 15° angle, stabilize the vein and penetrate the vein with one quick motion.

5. Pull back on the plunger of the syringe slowly until blood fills the syringe. Keep pulling slowly until you have obtained enough blood for the test(s) ordered.

6. Release the tourniquet, remove the needle from the patient's arm, apply pressure to the puncture site with a gauze square, and ask the patient to hold the gauze in place firmly with the arm straight.

7. Transfer blood to the evacuated tube(s) by inserting the needle through the rubber stopper and allowing the vacuum to pull the blood into the tube. To avoid a needle-stick injury, do not hold tubes while inserting the needle.

8. Gently rotate any tube(s) with additives and label.

9. When the bleeding has stopped, apply a bandage.

10. Remove gloves and discard in biohazard waste container, wash hands, and document.

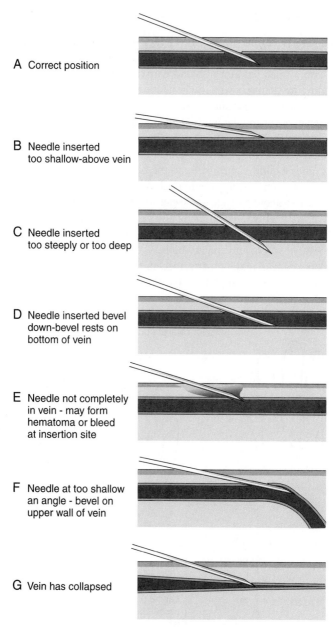

A Correct position

B Needle inserted
   too shallow-above vein

C Needle inserted
   too steeply or too deep

D Needle inserted bevel
   down-bevel rests on
   bottom of vein

E Needle not completely
   in vein - may form
   hematoma or bleed
   at insertion site

F Needle at too shallow
   an angle - bevel on
   upper wall of vein

G Vein has collapsed

FIGURE 10–3. Reasons for a failed blood draw.

CAPILLARY PUNCTURE

A capillary puncture is performed either on a finger (in older children and adults) or on a heel (in infants). Capillary punctures are performed to obtain a small amount of blood with which to perform blood tests, including frequent blood sugar tests for diabetic patients.

A diabetic patient, and often family members, must be taught how to perform a finger stick and test blood sugar using a glucometer.

Figure 10–4 shows sites for capillary punctures.

Heel sticks are performed on children who have not started to walk. Once a child begins to walk, the heel becomes callused and any capillary blood necessary should be drawn from the finger. Use the side of the heel to avoid damage to the calcaneus bone. Blood will flow more freely if the heel is warmed using a towel moistened with warm water for 5 to 10 minutes before the procedure. If necessary, the earlobe can also be used to obtain capillary blood.

A heel sticks may be performed in order to perform a phenylketonuria (PKU) test on a recently born baby. PKU is a metabolic

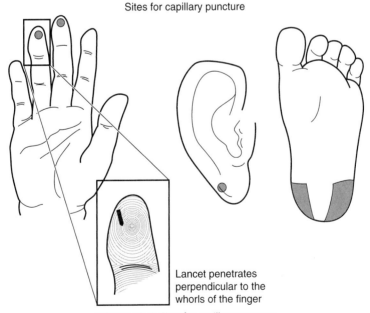

Sites for capillary puncture

Lancet penetrates
perpendicular to the
whorls of the finger

FIGURE 10–4. Sites for capillary puncture.

PROCEDURE FOR A FINGER STICK

1. Wash hands and assemble supplies.
2. Greet and identify patient, and explain the procedure.
3. Cleanse the finger selected for puncture using an alcohol pad.
4. Put on gloves.
5. Twist the small knot off a manual lancet, or prepare an automatic lancet.
6. Hold the finger in a downward position.
7. Without touching the area you have cleaned, make a puncture with the sterile lancet perpendicular to the fingerprint swirls on the lateral surface of the finger.
8. Drop lancet into sharps container.
9. Allow blood to flow. Wipe away the first drop of blood.
10. Collect a hanging drop of blood on pad of a test strip or collect a specimen in a microcollection device.
11. Place sterile gauze square over the puncture site and apply pressure. When the bleeding stops, apply bandage.
12. Perform tests.
13. Remove gloves and discard with soiled gauze in a biohazard waste container.
14. Wash hands; document.

condition in which an individual has a deleted gene that codes for phenylalanine hydroxylase. The person is unable to metabolize the amino acid phenylalanine, which is present in dairy and meat products. A special diet is necessary for infants who test positive for PKU.

THROAT SPECIMENS

Throat specimens are collected to test for group A beta hemolytic *Streptococcus* bacteria, the primary cause of bacterial pharyngitis (sore throat) in North America. Treating strep infections is important because untreated, strep infections can lead to bacterial endocarditis, rheumatic fever, or acute glomerulonephritis.

When collecting a throat culture:

- Use a tongue depressor to hold the tongue down.
- Use two long-stick sterile Dacron swabs.

- Obtain a specimen from the back of the throat without touching the tongue or teeth with the sterile swab.
- Swab the back of the throat in a figure-of-eight motion.
- Obtain the specimen from any visible pus on tonsils.

One swab may be used to perform a rapid strep test in the office. If that test is negative, the other swab will be either cultured in the office or sent to an outside lab to culture. To transport a specimen for culture, place the swab into a container with transport medium (such as a Culturette) and place the cap on the container. Squeeze the container firmly to release the transport medium, which will keep the specimen moist until it can be planted on a culture plate. Be sure to label the specimen and fill out any necessary requisition.

PROCEDURE FOR A HEEL STICK

1. Wash hands, assemble equipment, and open the alcohol pad and sterile gauze square.
2. Identify the infant, greet the infant's caregiver, and explain the procedure.
3. Warm the heel with a compress for a few minutes.
4. Clean the area of the heel where puncture will be made.
5. Put on gloves and prepare a pediatric lancet (which does not penetrate as deeply as an adult lancet).
6. Grasp the infant's heel firmly, and make the puncture on the side of the heel.
7. Dispose of the lancet in a rigid biohazard container.
8. Let blood flow, and wipe away first drop.
9. Collect specimen in appropriate microcollection container. If collecting a specimen to be tested for PKU, be sure that each circle of the test card is completely saturated with blood.
10. Place sterile gauze over puncture and apply pressure until bleeding stops; then cover with bandage.
11. Perform tests.
12. Remove gloves and dispose along with gauze in biohazard waste container.
13. Wash hands; document.

WOUND SPECIMENS

A wound may contain aerobic or anaerobic bacteria. Deep wounds especially are likely to contain anaerobic bacteria, which flourish under conditions with no oxygen.

Wound specimens should be collected from the wound (not the dressing) before cleaning and redressing the wound. Sterile gloves should be worn to collect the specimens.

Be sure that the doctor sees any wound that has exudate or drainage, and use a sterile swab to collect a specimen from any wound that appears to be infected, when ordered.

First, use a swab from an anaerobic culture kit and collect a specimen from the deepest part of the wound. Then use a swab from an aerobic culture kit and collect a specimen from the surface where the most exudate is present.

Each swab is placed in an culture tube immediately, and the media-transport ampule should be crushed by squeezing the sides of the tube firmly.

After specimens have been taken, change gloves and clean and redress the wound. Then discard all the waste in the biohazard waste container, remove and discard gloves, wash hands, and document.

URINE SPECIMENS

Urine specimens can be collected in a number of different ways, for many different purposes. There are:

- Random urine specimens
- Clean-catch midstream specimens
- First morning specimens
- 24-hour specimens
- Specimens for drug testing

Random Urine Specimen

Random urine specimens are used for pregnancy-confirmation tests and general tests as part of a routine physical.

To collect a random sample, label a specimen cup, instruct the patient to void approximately 50 to 100 mL of urine into the specimen cup, and replace the cover tightly. Wear gloves to handle the specimen.

Clean-Catch Midstream

A clean-catch midstream specimen is the method of choice for microscopic examination, as well as for pregnancy testing and urinalysis.

To obtain a clean-catch midstream sample, you need to instruct the patient in how to properly clean his or her genital area and collect the urine without contaminating the collection device. Instruct the patient to wash hands before collecting the urine specimen and avoid touching the inside of the lid or container. Tell the patient where to take or leave the specimen.

Collection procedure for females:

1. Spread the labia and clean the genital area from front to back using each cleansing towel only once.
2. Continue to hold the labia apart and void a small amount into the toilet. Then void into the specimen cup until it is about half-full and void any remaining urine into the toilet.
3. Replace the lid without touching the inside of the lid or container.
4. Wash hands after collection is complete.

Collection procedure for males:

1. Retract the foreskin of the penis (if uncircumcised) and cleanse the glans using each cleansing towel once.
2. Holding the foreskin retracted, void a small amount into the toilet. Then void into the specimen cup until it is about half-full and void any remaining urine into the toilet.
3. Replace the cover without touching the inside of the cover or the specimen cup.
4. Wash hands after collection is complete.

First Morning Urine Specimen

The first morning void is a concentrated specimen and is often used to test for urine chemicals, such as nitrites. Unless the patient is hospitalized, the first morning void needs to be collected at home by the patient. Again, you must give the patient instructions on proper collection and delivery for testing or proper storage.

24-Hour Sample

The 24-hour urine collection is again most often done by the patient. You must give the patient proper instructions as to collecting and proper storage (refrigeration) of the sample during the 24-hour period. Depending on the substance to be tested, you may need to add a preservative to the collection bottle. If a preservative is used, the patient should not void directly into the 24-hour collection container.

Give the patient the following instructions:

1. Avoid alcoholic beverages, vitamins, and over-the-counter medications for at least 24 hours before and during specimen collection.
2. Refrain from emptying the bottle before starting the test and avoid contact with any chemical in the bottle.
3. Keep the container out of the reach of children.
4. Keep the collection bottle in a cool place, preferably in the refrigerator.
5. Collect the urine on a day that you will be able to collect all urine (each time you void) and bring it to the collection facility promptly when specimen collection is complete.
6. Begin this test in the morning. Do not collect the first morning specimen. Void the first time that day into the toilet and flush. Note the time and date of this void on the container.
7. Collect all urine specimens for the next 24 hours. Collect the specimens in a urinal (males) or toilet insert (females) and pour into the collection bottle using a funnel. The final collection includes the first morning void the next morning.
8. Do not put anything except urine into the container (e.g., toilet paper, stool, tampons, and so on).
9. Do not dip urine from the toilet bowl because it will be diluted with water.
10. Call the office if you have questions or concerns.
11. Return the specimen to the laboratory the morning the test is completed.

Specimens for Drug Testing

Sometimes a urine specimen is collected for drug testing. A drug-screen urine sample is essentially a random sample. Proper documentation must be prepared and special steps taken to preserve the "chain of custody" of the sample.

Often, an individual providing a specimen for drug testing is observed or allowed to wear only a gown and placed in a bathroom facility where clear water is not available. A seal is placed over the specimen container cap, and it is initialed by the individual who

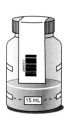
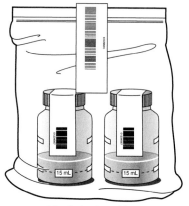

Urine bottle sealed
with barcode label

Plastic transport bag
sealed with barcode label

FIGURE 10–5. Urine specimens for drug screening are sealed with bar-coded labels to prevent tampering after collection.

performed the test or instructed the patient and collected and sealed the sample as shown in Figure 10–5.

Every individual from that point on who handles the specimen must initial the documentation and must physically hand the specimen to the next person who will be responsible for it.

FECAL SPECIMENS

Fecal samples are taken for one of two reasons:

- In a routine physical exam, a fecal matter smear is taken on a gloved finger during the rectal exam. This fecal sample is tested for the presence of occult (hidden) blood using a fecal blood test kit. You may help the doctor by assembling the proper supplies, or you may be asked to perform the test.
- A fecal sample is also taken for a patient suffering from a diarrheal illness and sent to a laboratory for testing for the presence of parasites or parasite ova. In this instance, you may need to instruct the patient on how to take a fecal sample at home and provide gloves. The patient should place a film of plastic wrap over the surface of the toilet to avoid having the stool become wet. A portion of the stool should be placed in a container with a tight lid and transported to the laboratory as soon as possible to avoid a

change in the pH of the specimen that could cause death of the parasites or ova.

SPUTUM SPECIMENS

A sputum sample is used to diagnose infectious diseases of the respiratory tract, such as tuberculosis or pneumonia. You may be asked to collect a sputum sample or assist in collecting a sputum sample, using one of three methods:

- Expectoration, in which the patient coughs up mucus and spits it into a collection cup
- Suctioning, in which a sterile catheter is passed into the trachea to collect such mucus from the trachea and lungs
- Bronchoscopy, in which a physician places a bronchoscope into the patient's trachea and collects sputum with a bronchial brush

When collecting a sputum sample, always wear:

- Gloves
- Mask
- Goggles or face shield
- Gown

Label the specimen and complete any requisition before sending the specimen to the laboratory.

Chapter 11

Diagnostic Testing

As a medical assistant, you will be asked to perform some diagnostic tests; assist with other tests; collect, label, and transport samples for other tests; and provide patients with instructions on how to prepare for other tests.

This chapter reviews common laboratory tests you are able to do yourself and gives some information about instructing patients for tests done outside the office.

QUALITY CONTROL

Quality control is the process used to ensure the validity and accuracy of test results. Quality control involves monitoring proficiency of employees and performing daily calibration of equipment. It also includes tests (called controls) to measure the precision of instrumentation and the quality of the chemicals and reagents used in order to ensure accuracy of test results.

Quality control identifies human error in procedures, problems with chemicals or reagents used in test kits, and automated testing equipment that is not performing as expected. Preventive maintenance of laboratory equipment is also an integral part of quality control.

Records of all quality control activities must be kept, including:

- Specimen identification
- Reagent, chemical, and instrumentation test results
- Instrument maintenance history

URINALYSIS

The urine dipstick is the most common testing methodology used in the medical office to test the chemical properties of urine.

Reagent strips (called dipsticks) are used to detect urine chemicals. Dipsticks determine how much of a substance is present in urine (quantitative testing) based on the color changes that occur, which are easy to interpret. Dipstick testing can use either manual or automated testing equipment to provide results.

Urine reagent strip tests can be used to determine if the following substances are present in urine:

- Blood
- Leukocytes
- Nitrites
- Protein
- Glucose and ketones
- Bilirubin and urobilinogen

They are also used to test the pH and specific gravity of urine.

PROCEDURE FOR URINALYSIS USING A REAGENT STRIP

1. Wash hands.
2. Assemble necessary supplies. These include a vial of urine reagent dipsticks (e.g., Multistix 10 or Chemstix); clean, dry gauze pads; a timer that measures seconds and minutes; and a fresh, well-mixed urine specimen.
3. Put on disposable gloves.
4. Be sure controls have been run for the day.
5. Open bottle of strips and remove one. Close the bottle immediately to prevent deterioration of the remaining strips.
6. Quickly dip the strip into the urine specimen, completely immersing the strip.
7. Remove the strip and hold it horizontally so it does not drip from one pad to another.
8. Blot the strip on gauze, making sure the reagent pads do not touch the gauze.

(continued)

PROCEDURE FOR URINALYSIS USING A REAGENT STRIP *Continued*

9. Set timer according to manufacturer's specifications.
10. At specified time, compare colors of the various pads to the color chart provided. Mentally note any abnormal results.
11. Dispose of strip, gloves, and unused specimen in biohazard waste container.
12. Wash hands.
13. Document results. Also document the color and turbidity of the specimen.

HEMATOLOGIC TESTING

Hematologic testing includes tests such as the following:

- Complete blood count (CBC) with or without differential cell count (diff)
- Hemoglobin determination (Hgb)
- Microhematocrit (Hct)
- Erythrocyte sedimentation rate (ESR)

The complete blood count includes:

- White blood cell (WBC) count
- Red blood cell (RBC) count
- Platelet count
- RBC indices, which are used to determine different kinds of anemia
- Hematocrit (percentage of packed RBCs)
- Hemoglobin level
- An optional differential WBC count, which identifies the percentage of each type of WBC present in the sample.

The reference ranges for a complete blood count are shown in Table 11–1.

CHEMISTRY TESTING

Blood is usually drawn in the office for blood chemistry testing to be done at an outside laboratory. If more than one test is to be done, the

TABLE 11-1
Reference Ranges for Complete Blood Count and Differential

Test	Neonates	Infants to 6 mo	Children	Adult Men	Adult Women
WBC	9–30 × 1000/mm³	6–16 × 1000/mm³	5–12 × 1000/mm³	4.5–11.0 × 1000/mm³	4.5–11.0 × 1000/mm³
RBC	4.8–7.0 million/mm³	3.8–5.5 million/mm³	4.5–4.8 million/mm³	4.6–6.2 million/mm³	2.4–5.4 million/mm³
MCV	96–108 μm	—	—	82–98 μm	82–98 μm
MCH	32–24 pg	—	—	26–34 pg	26–24 pg
MCHC	31–33 g/dL	—	—	31–33 g/dL	31–33 g/dL
Platelets	140–300 × 1000/mm³	200–475 × 1000/mm³	150–450 × 1000/mm³	150–400 × 1000/mm³	150–400 × 1000/mm³
Differential					
Neutrophils	—	—	—	50–60%	50–60%
Bands	—	—	—	0–3%	0–3%
Eosinophils	—	—	—	1–3%	1–3%
Basophils	—	—	—	0–3%	0–3%
Monocytes	—	—	—	4–9%	4–9%
Lymphocytes	—	—	—	25–40%	25–40%

PROCEDURE FOR TESTING HEMOGLOBIN USING A HEMOGLOBINOMETER

1. Wash hands.
2. Assemble supplies and equipment. Prepare the hemoglobinometer by removing the chamber and opening it so the chamber slide is visible.
3. Put on gloves.
4. Perform a finger stick and wipe away the first drop of blood (or remove small amount of blood from a venous blood sample collected in a tube with a lavender stopper).
5. Place drop of blood into the chamber slide.
6. Use a wooden stick to stir the drop of blood for about 45 seconds to hemolyze the RBCs.
7. Close the chamber slide and insert it into the hemoglobinometer.
8. Hold the device at eye level and turn on the light.
9. Look through eyepiece. Move the slide on the right of the instrument until both sides of the split field appear to be the same shade of green.
10. Read the scale on the side of the instrument to identify the hemoglobin reading in grams per deciliter of blood.
11. Record results, then clean area and device, and dispose of materials and gloves in appropriate biohazard waste containers.

PROCEDURE TO TEST MICROHEMATOCRIT

1. Wash hands.
2. Assemble supplies and equipment, including capillary tubes and sealing clay. If performing a finger stick, the capillary tube should be heparinized.
3. Put on gloves.
4. Obtain a venous or capillary blood sample or use blood from a venous sample taken from a sample collected in a tube with a lavender stopper. You need enough blood to fill two capillary tubes three quarters full.
5. Seal one end of each tube with clay sealant.
6. Place tubes opposite each other in microhematocrit centrifuge, clay sealant end out.

PROCEDURE TO TEST MICROHEMATOCRIT *Continued*

7. Set timer to just past 5 minutes.
8. After centrifuge has completely stopped, remove lid.
9. Remove the two tubes carefully.
10. Align the top of the clay sealant, where RBCs begin, to the "0" mark on the microhematocrit reader.
11. Move the outer disk until the reading line is directly under the junction of the packed RBCs and the buffy coat. Read the result on the scale at the outer edge of the reader.
12. Average the readings from the two tubes.
13. Discard the tubes in a sharps container and the other materials and gloves in a biohazard waste container.
14. Wash hands and document results.

---

patient is charged for a blood chemistry panel, a set of related chemistry tests, such as a liver panel, a cardiac panel, or a chemistry screen.

Table 11–2 shows blood chemistry normal values.

The most common blood chemistry test performed in the office is a blood glucose test using a glucometer. Elevated blood glucose (hyperglycemia) is associated with diabetes mellitus. However, devices similar to a glucometer may be used to test blood cholesterol or other substances in the office.

TABLE 11–2
Blood Chemistry Normal Values

Name of Test	Abbreviation	Reference Range for Adults
Alanine aminotransferase	ALT	6–37 U/L
Albumin	—	3.5–5.5 g/dL
Alkaline phosphatase	ALP	0.8–2.0 BLB Unit
Amylase	—	95–290 U/L
Anion gap (R factor)	AG	10–18 mEq/L
Aspartate transaminase	AST	5–30 U/L
Bilirubin, conjugated	—	0.1–0.3 mg/dL
Bilirubin, total	—	0.2–1.0 mg/dL

(continued)

TABLE 11–2
Blood Chemistry Normal Values *Continued*

Name of Test	Abbreviation	Reference Range for Adults
Blood urea nitrogen	BUN	5–20 mg/dL
Calcium	Ca	8.4–10.2 mg/dL
Carbon dioxide	CO_2	22–29 mEq/L
Chloride	Cl	98–106 mmol/L
Cholesterol, total	CH or Chol	Desirable: <200 mg/dL Borderline: 200–239 mg/dL High: >240 mg/dL
Low-density lipoprotein	LDL	Desirable: <170 mg/dL Borderline: 170–199 mg/dL High: >200 mg/dL
High-density lipoprotein	HDL	Males: 29–60 mg/dL Females: 38–75 mg/dL
Creatine kinase	CK	Males: 15–160 U/L Females: 15–130 U/L
Creatinine	—	Males: 0.6–1.2 mg/dL Females: 0.5–1.1 mg/dL
Glucose, fasting	FBS	70–100 mg/dL
Glucose, 2 h postprandial	PPBS	<140 mg/dL
Glucose tolerance test	GTT	FBS: 70–110 mg/dL 30 min: 110–170 mg/dL 1 h: 120–170 mg/dL 2 h: 70–120 mg/dL 3 h: <120 mg/dL
Iron	Fe	40–160 µg/dL
Total iron binding capacity	TIBC	250–400 µg/dL
Lactic dehydrogenase	LD	100–200 U/L
Lipase	—	0–1.0 U/mL
Magnesium	Mag, Mg	1.3–2.1 mEq/L
Phosphorus	P	2.7–4.5 mg/dL
Potassium	K	3.5–5.1 mEq/L
Protein, total	TP	6.2–8.2 g dL
Sodium	Na	136–146 mEq/L
Triglycerides	Trig	10–190 mg/dL
Uric acid	—	Males: 3.5–7.2 mg/dL Females: 2.6–6.0 mg/dL

PROCEDURE TO TEST BLOOD GLUCOSE USING A GLUCOMETER ELITE ANALYZER

1. Wash hands.
2. Assemble equipment and supplies, which include gloves, Glucometer Elite Analyzer, batteries, check strip, code strip for calibration, test strips, glucose control normal level, lancet, gauze, bandage, and alcohol pads.
3. Use check strip to check meter performance, following manufacturer's instructions.
4. Calibrate instrument with code strip for new batch of test strips, if necessary.
5. Wash hands again.
6. Identify and greet patient, and explain procedure.
7. Put on gloves.
8. Hold the test end of a new strip between two layers of foil and insert fully into the meter. Listen for beep, followed by function number on display screen.
9. Perform finger stick.
10. Wipe away first drop of blood, and touch test end of strip to the second drop of blood until a beep is heard.
11. Result will appear after 59 seconds and will be stored when strip is removed.
12. Dispose of gloves and supplies in appropriate biohazard waste containers, wash hands, and record results.

IMMUNOLOGY TESTING

Immunology tests use antibodies to specific proteins to test for particular conditions, or tests that determine if antibodies are present in a specimen. Some immunology tests require serum specimens, while others are conducted on urine. The rapid test for streptococcal sore throat is also an immunology test.

Among the most frequently performed immunology tests are blood tests for mononucleosis, tests for *Streptococcus* A, tests for *H. pylori*, and urine pregnancy tests.

PROCEDURE TO PERFORM A URINE PREGNANCY TEST

1. Wash hands.
2. Assemble supplies.
3. Put on disposable gloves.
4. Open a pregnancy test kit.
5. Aspirate urine with disposable pipette.
6. Drop three drops of urine in the test well.
7. Time for 3 minutes (or as directed by manufacturer), then check indicator and note if the test is positive or negative.
8. Dispose of gloves and supplies in appropriate biohazard waste container.
9. Wash hands and record date, time, results, and brand of test used.

PROCEDURE TO TEST THROAT CULTURE SPECIMEN FOR *STREPTOCOCCUS* A

1. Wash hands.
2. Assemble supplies and equipment, including throat culture specimen, test kit with reagents.
3. Put on disposable gloves.
4. Place open plastic tube in test kit tube holder.
5. Place the number of drops of reagents in the test tube as specified by the manufacturer.
6. Place one specimen swab in the tube and mix well. Allow swab to stay in tube for 2 to 15 minutes (or as specified by manufacturer).
7. Add the number of drops of additional reagent(s) specified by the manufacturer.
8. Use swab to mix all contents.
9. Roll swab head against side of tube to express all contents from the swab.
10. Put cap on tube and perform test within 1 hour or perform test immediately.

PROCEDURE TO TEST THROAT CULTURE SPECIMEN FOR *STREPTOCOCCUS* A *Continued*

11. Drop three drops on the paper in the sample window of the test unit, and begin timing. Read in 5 minutes or as specified by the manufacturer.
12. If result is negative, follow up with traditional throat culture.
13. Dispose of gloves and materials in proper biohazard containers, wash hands, and document results.

MICROBIOLOGY TESTING

Microbiology tests use a microscope to look for organisms present in samples. Samples are placed on a slide or on a culture plate with agar or another growth medium to see if bacteria grow in the sample.

Figure 11–1 (p. 139) illustrates planting a specimen on an agar plate.

PROCEDURE TO PREPARE A WET MOUNT HANGING DROP SLIDE

1. Wash hands.
2. Assemble glass slides, cover slip, petroleum jelly, sample to be examined, microscope, and disposable gloves.
3. Put on disposable gloves.
4. Place petroleum jelly around the edge of a cover slip.
5. Place a drop of solution containing material to be examined on the cover slip.
6. Place a hanging drop slide over the cover slip so the depression in the slide is centered over the drop of solution.
7. Apply pressure to fix the cover slip to the slide.
8. Turn the slide over quickly so the drop of solution hangs from the cover slip into the slide well.
9. Place the slide on the microscope.
10. Dispose of materials and gloves in the proper biohazard waste containers.

PROCEDURE TO PLANT, OR "INOCULATE," A CULTURE ON AN AGAR PLATE

1. Wash hands.
2. Assemble supplies and equipment, including loop incinerator and metal loop (or disposable loops), loop holder, specimen on swab(s), blood agar plate, and marker.
3. Turn on loop incinerator; place loop in loop holder where you will be working (if using reusable loop).
4. Put on gloves and face protection.
5. Place a blood agar plate on the counter, agar side down, and remove cover.
6. Take one specimen swab and streak approximately one quarter of the agar plate with the swab.
7. Flame the inoculation loop, or remove a disposable loop from package.
8. Going into the streak at right angles, use loop to spread the specimen into the second quadrant of plate.
9. Reflame the loop or use another disposable loop to go into the streak again and spread to the third quadrant, then again into the remainder of the plate. Reflame the reusable loop again at end of the process, and turn off the incinerator.
10. Replace the cover on the agar plate and label the specimen. Put the plate in the incubator, agar side up to prevent drips from condensation, or place the specimen in a biohazard transport bag with appropriate documentation. If incubating in the office, record the source of the specimen and time and date placed in the incubator in the laboratory log.
11. Dispose of gloves and materials in appropriate biohazard containers, wash hands, and complete necessary documentation.

1. First quadrant-swab

2. Second quadrant-loop

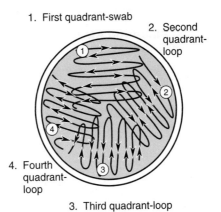

4. Fourth quadrant-loop

3. Third quadrant-loop

FIGURE 11–1. Illustration of method to plant a specimen on an agar plate.

ELECTROCARDIOGRAPHY

Electrocardiography (ECG) is the visual recording of the heart's electrical activity using a set of electrodes attached to a patient's skin to conduct electricity. The ECG machine records electrical activity from various combinations of electrodes called leads. The pattern, called a tracing, records the electrical activity of all parts of the heart so the doctor can draw conclusions about how effectively the heart is working.

PROCEDURE TO PERFORM AN ELECTROCARDIOGRAM

1. Check to make sure machine is set up correctly and turn the machine on to warm up.
2. Identify and greet patient, explain the purpose of the test, and explain that the patient must lie still without talking during the test.
3. Instruct a male to remove his shirt and a female to undress from the waist up and put on a gown with the opening in the front. Provide privacy.
4. Wash hands.

(continued)

PROCEDURE TO PERFORM AN
ELECTROCARDIOGRAM *Continued*

5. Position the patient resting comfortably in the supine position. The area where tabs or electrodes will be placed should be clean and dry.

6. Place electrodes tab-down on the arms and chest, and tabs facing up on the legs, and attach the correct cable to each electrode.

7. Place electrodes on the chest tab-down following the lead-placement guide shown in Figure 11–2, and attach the correct cable to each electrode.

8. Instruct the patient to lie still, and press the auto button to run the tracing. Observe the tracing to be sure the tracing is clear.

9. Remove electrodes from the patient and store the patient cable neatly on the machine.

10. Label the ECG with the patient's name, date, age, cardiac symptoms, and cardiac medications. If using a single-channel machine, mount the tracing. Place the ECG for the physician to review.

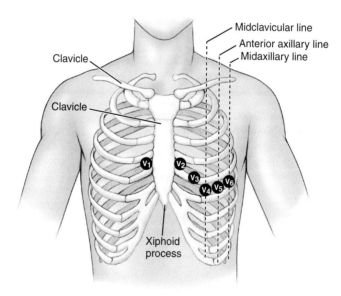

FIGURE 11–2. Placement of chest electrodes for an electrocardiogram.

PROCEDURE TO PERFORM SPIROMETRY *Continued*

11. Discard mouthpiece, nose clip (if used), and tubing in biohazard waste container.
12. Wash hands; place documentation in the patient's file.

Urinary Catheterization

You will probably be asked only to catheterize a female patient, although you may be asked to prepare the equipment for a doctor to catheterize a male patient.

PROCEDURE FOR CATHETERIZING A FEMALE PATIENT

1. Wash hands.
2. Assemble equipment, including a catheter tray with a sterile catheter, sterile gloves, sterile cotton balls, sterile forceps, solution for cleaning, lubricant, and sterile towels for draping the patient.
3. Identify and greet the patient, and explain the procedure.
4. Have the patient undress from the waist down and lie on the exam table in the dorsal recumbent position. Pull out the table extension to support the patient's feet.
5. Verify that the patient is not allergic to povidone–iodine (Betadine) or shellfish.
6. Open disposable sterile kit using sterile technique and create a sterile field. Place the drape over the patient, leaving the perineal area open and touching only the edges of the drape.
7. Put on sterile gloves.
8. Pour povidone–iodine over the cotton balls and lubricate 2 to 3 inches of the catheter tip. Place the tray container nearby to hold urine, and open the specimen container and place nearby.
9. Inform the patient before you begin the actual procedure.
10. With nondominant hand, spread labia as wide as possible to expose urethra and urethral meatus. Do not allow labia to fall back together until the catheter has been used and removed. See Figure 11–4 for an illustration of this step.

(continued)

PROCEDURE FOR CATHETERIZING A FEMALE PATIENT *Continued*

11. Pick up one cotton ball with forceps and, using one motion, swipe down on one side of labia, then discard cotton ball. Repeat on the other side. Repeat down the middle.

12. With dominant hand, pick up the lubricated catheter and tell the patient you are about to insert the catheter.

13. Insert catheter about 2 to 3 inches until urine begins to flow. Let some urine flow into the overflow container, then catch some urine in the sterile collection container. When the specimen container is full, allow the remaining urine to flow into the overflow container.

(continued)

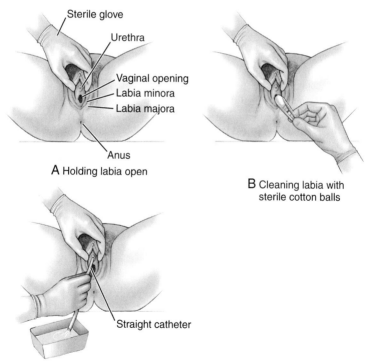

A Holding labia open

B Cleaning labia with sterile cotton balls

C Collecting urine from straight catheter

FIGURE 11–4. Female catheterization. *A,* Holding labia open. *B,* Cleaning labia with sterile cotton balls. *C,* Collecting urine from a straight catheter.

PROCEDURE FOR CATHETERIZING A FEMALE PATIENT *Continued*

14. When the urine stops flowing, remove the catheter, place the lid on the specimen container, and clean the patient. Once the catheter has been removed, sterile technique is no longer necessary.
15. Place specimen container in a biohazard transport bag.
16. Measure the amount of urine and discard. Discard supplies and gloves in biohazard waste container.
17. Wash hands and document the procedure, including the amount of urine obtained and the type of specimen tested or sent to the laboratory.

Diagnostic Imaging

Diagnostic imaging uses a number of various imaging devices, from plain-film x-rays to sophisticated nuclear medicine, computed tomography (CT), and magnetic resonance imaging (MRI). Table 11–3 summarizes information about various modalities used to create images to facilitate diagnosis.

Plain-film x-rays are still the most commonly used diagnostic imaging. When ordering x-rays, the doctor will order that the patient be placed in specific positions so the x-ray will show the body at one of four angles, using one of four projections:

- Anteroposterior (front to back)
- Posteroanterior (back to front)
- Lateral (side to side)
- Oblique (at an angle)

The patient positions for these four types of images are shown in Figure 11–5 (pp. 147–148).

You will be asked to provide instructions to the patient about where to go to obtain the appropriate diagnostic imagine study and any special preparations for the study.

The medical assistant may schedule diagnostic tests and provide instructions to patients before the test. The process of instructing patients is described in more detail in Chapter 16, Patient Instruction. You should find out where to schedule tests and where the instruction sheets for patients are kept. Be sure to ask a female patient if there is any possibility that she could be pregnant before scheduling an x-ray or CT scan (which uses x-rays). Days 1 to 10 of the menstrual cycle are considered to be a safe time to take x-rays in a woman who is fertile and sexually active.

TABLE 11–3 Modalities Used for Diagnostic Imaging	
Modality	**Description**
Diagnostic radiology	Uses x-ray to form a diagnostic image
Fluoroscopy	Continuous x-ray imaging; usually used when studies require swallowing a contrast material (e.g., barium) or placement of a catheter within an artery to inject contrast material
Tomography	Creation of a series of cross-sectional images
Computed tomography (CT)	Linking cross-sectional images using a computer; may be done with or without injection of a contrast material
Magnetic resonance imaging (MRI)	Uses magnetic fields in combination with radio waves and computer technology to create cross-sectional views of tissue
Nuclear medicine	A process of diagnostic imaging using radioactive material injected into the patient or swallowed by the patient and followed by a scan of various body parts to detect uptake of the radioactive material by body tissue; the scan is often named for the radioactive material (e.g., gallium scan, thallium scan)
Diagnostic medical sonography (ultrasound)	Uses ultrasound (inaudible high frequency sound waves) to form a diagnostic image; ultrasonic waves directed toward the body form echoes whose varying densities give information about underlying structures

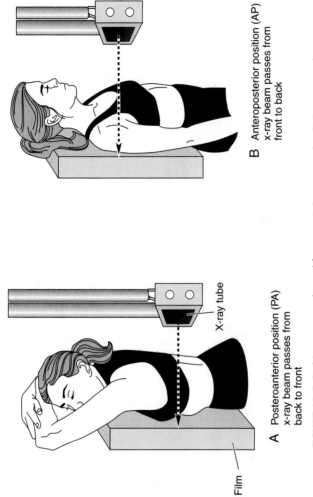

FIGURE 11–5. Positions commonly used for x-ray. *A*, Posteroanterior. *B*, Anteroposterior.

Figure continued on following page

A Posteroanterior position (PA)
x-ray beam passes from
back to front

X-ray tube

Film

B Anteroposterior position (AP)
x-ray beam passes from
front to back

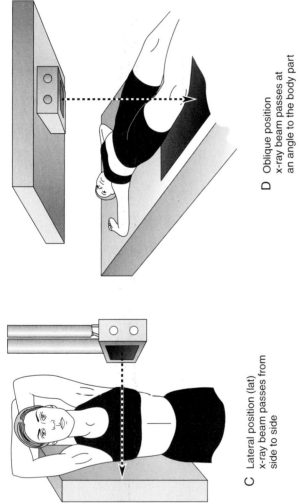

C Lateral position (lat)
   x-ray beam passes from
   side to side

D Oblique position
   x-ray beam passes at
   an angle to the body part

FIGURE 11-5 *Continued. C,* Lateral. *D,* Oblique.

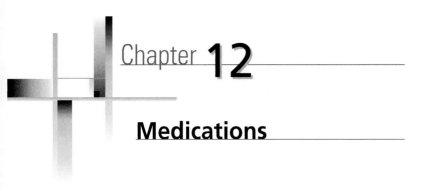

Chapter 12

Medications

ABOUT MEDICATION ADMINISTRATION

In many states, medical assistants are able to give medications in the medical office. Because medication administration can pose a risk to any patient, the medical assistant must always be careful to follow the correct procedure and take all possible measures to prevent injury or adverse effects. **Because the medical assistant is not specifically licensed to administer medications in most states, he or she should never give a patient a dose of a medication unless the physician is present in the office to respond to any problem or adverse effect.**

MEDICATION CALCULATIONS

Before preparing a medication, it is often necessary to calculate the correct dose. Any medication calculation can be expressed as a proportion, where the unknown (x) is the amount to give. Refer to Table 12–1 (p. 150) if you need to review abbreviations used in calculating and preparing medications.

Calculating Dose of Solid Medication

In the case of a solid medication, usually you know the dose per tablet or capsule from the doctor's orders. x is the number of tablets or capsules to give. The equation is:

$$\frac{\text{dose ordered}}{\text{dose per unit (tablet, capsule)}} = x \text{ units}$$

TABLE 12–1
Common Abbreviations Used for Ordering and
Administering Medications

ac	before meals	NKA	no known allergies
AD	right ear	noc, noct	night
ad lib	as desired	npo, NPO	nothing by mouth
am, AM	morning	NS	normal saline
amp	ampule	OD	right eye
amt	amount	ophth	ophthalmic
AS	left ear	os	mouth
aq	aqueous	OS	left eye
AU	both ears	OU	both eyes
bid	twice a day	oz, $\overline{3}$	ounce
$\overline{c}$	with	$\overline{p}$	after
cap	capsule	pc	after meals
DC, disc, d/c	discontinue	po, PO	by mouth
dr, $\overline{3}$	dram	pm, PM	afternoon
DW	distilled water	prn, PRN	as needed
elix	elixir	pt	patient or pint
et	and	q	every
ext	extract	qd	every day
fl	fluid	q 2 h	every 2 hours
g	gram	qid	four times a day
gr	grain	qs	quantity sufficient
gt(t)	drop(s)	Rx	take, prescribe
h, hr	hour	$\overline{s}$	without
hs, HS	hour of sleep	SC, subq, S/Q	subcutaneous
ID	intradermal	Sig	directions to patient
IM	intramuscular	sl, SL	sublingual
IU	international units	sol	solution
IV	intravenous	ss, $\overline{ss}$	half
kg	kilogram	stat, STAT	immediately
L	liter	supp	suppository
lb	pound	T, Tbsp	tablespoon
m, min, $\mathfrak{M}$	minim	t, tsp	teaspoon
mcg, μg	microgram	tab	tablet
mEq	milliequivalent	tid	three times a day
mg	milligram	tinc, tinct	tincture
mL	milliliter	ung	ointment
NaCl	sodium chloride	U	units

For instance, the doctor orders 750 mg of the antibiotic ciprofloxacin (Cipro). Cipro comes in 250-mg tablets. The equation to calculate the correct dose to give is:

$$\frac{750 \text{ mg}}{250 \text{ mg/tablet}} = 3 \text{ tablets}$$

Remember, to solve a fraction, divide the bottom number into the top number.

Calculating a Dose of Liquid Medication

When a liquid medication is expressed in a unit of one (e.g., per teaspoon), the equation can be solved the same way as for a solid medication.

When a liquid medication is expressed in units other than one, the calculation is more complex. There are two ways to solve such an equation: a two-step method and a one-step method.

For instance, the doctor has ordered erythromycin, oral suspension, 250 mg. The label on the bottle says there are 125 mg per 5 mL.

Two-Step Calculation

Step 1. Calculate the number of milligrams in 1 mL by dividing 5 into 125.

$$\frac{125 \text{ mg}}{5 \text{ mL}} = \frac{25 \text{ mg}}{1 \text{ mL}}$$

Step 2. Using the number of milligrams per milliliter, calculate the desired dose, setting up the fraction with the dose ordered over the dose per milliliter:

$$\frac{250 \text{ mg}}{25 \text{ mg/mL}} = 10 \text{ mL}$$

The desired dose, or amount to give the patient, is 10 mL.

One-Step Calculation

Use the following formula to find the dose using only one calculation. Remember that parentheses in a formula mean that you should multiply.

TABLE 12–2 Prefixes Used in the Metric System						
Latin Prefixes			*No Prefix*	*Greek Prefixes*		
micro-	milli-	deci-	**none**	deca-	hecto-	kilo-
0.000001	0.001	0.1	**1**	10	100	1000
millionth	thousandth	tenth	**one**	ten	hundred	thousand

$$\frac{\text{(dose ordered by weight)(quantity or volume)}}{\text{dose on hand (by weight)}} = \text{amount to give}$$

For the problem at hand, the equation is:

$$\frac{250 \text{ mg} \times 5 \text{ mL}}{125 \text{ mg}} = \frac{1250 \text{ mg} \times \text{mL}}{125 \text{ mg}} = 10 \text{ mL}$$

As in the two-step method, you should give 10 mL of the medication.

If you need to review prefixes in the metric system, see Table 12–2. For conversion tables for the apothecaries', household, and metric systems, see Table 12–3.

Pediatric Doses

You can calculate a pediatric dose using either body weight or body surface area (BSA). To calculate a pediatric dose by body weight (expressed in kilograms), use the following three-step procedure.

Step 1. Calculate the number of kilograms in the child's weight. The conversion formula is 2.2 lb = 1 kg. To change pounds to kilograms, divide by 2.2.

Step 2. Calculate the number of milligrams to give each day.

Step 3. Calculate the number of milligrams to give with each dose.

For example, a doctor orders medication for a child at 10 mg/kg, to be given in two doses. The child weighs 75 lb.

Step 1. 75 lb = x kg

$$\frac{75}{2.2} = 34 \text{ kg}$$

TABLE 12–3
Conversion Tables for Apothecaries', Household, and Metric Measurements

Apothecaries'/Metric Units of Weight*

Apothecaries'	Metric
gr 1/60 (one sixtieth of a grain)	1 mg
gr 1/30	2 mg
gr 1/20	3 mg
gr 1/15	4 mg
gr 1/10	6 mg
gr 1/6	10 mg
gr ¼	15 mg
gr ½	30 mg
gr i (1 grain)	60 mg
gr v (5 grains)	300 mg
gr x (10 grains)	600 mg
gr 15	1000 mg
dr i (60 grains = 1 dram)	4 g

Household (Avoirdupois)/Metric Units of Weight

Household	Metric
1 oz	30 g
1 lb (1 lb = 16 oz)	454 g
2.2 lb	1 kg

Apothecaries'/Household/Metric Units of Volume†

Apothecaries'	Household	Metric
min i (1 minim)	gt i (1 drop)	0.06 mL
min xv (15 minims)	tsp ss (½ tsp)	—
min 16	—	1 mL (1 cc)
fl dr i (1 fluidram)	tsp i (1 tsp)	5 mL (5 cc)
fl oz i (1 fluid oz)	Tbsp ii (3 tsp = 1 Tbsp)	30 mL (30 cc)
fl oz iv	—	120 mL (120 cc)
fl oz viii	1 cup	—
fl oz 16	1 pint	500 mL (500 cc)

*For easier calculation, a grain is commonly considered to be 60 mg instead of 65 mg in conversion tables. This means that a 5-gr tablet of aspirin or acetaminophen actually contains 325 mg of medication.
†The conversion equivalents used for liquid measurement are also approximate for ease in calculation.

Step 2. $(34 \text{ kg})(10 \text{ mg/kg}) = x \text{ mg/day}$

$$(34)(10) = 340 \text{ mg/day}$$

Step 3. 340 mg divided by 2 doses $= x$ mg/dose

$$\frac{340}{2} = 170 \text{ mg/dose}$$

To calculate a pediatric dose using the BSA method, the dose is expressed in terms of the child's BSA, in square meters (m^2). The equation is:

$$\text{Child dose} = \frac{\text{BSA (in m}^2\text{)}}{1.7 \text{ m}^2} \times (\text{adult dose})$$

To calculate the child's BSA, draw a line connecting the child's height and weight on the nomogram shown in Figure 12–1.

Example: Judy is a 4-year-old girl who is 41 inches tall and weighs 35 lb. As you can validate from Figure 12–1, her BSA is 0.69 m^2. What is the correct dose of erythromycin if the usual adult dose is 250 mg?
Step 1:

$$\frac{0.69 \text{ m}^2}{1.7 \text{ m}^2} \times (250 \text{ mg}) = x \text{ mg (correct dose)}$$

Step 2:

$$\frac{(0.69 \text{ m}^2)(250 \text{ mg})}{1.7 \text{ m}^2} = \frac{175.2 \text{ mg}}{1.7} \approx 101 \text{ mg (correct dose)}$$

Five Rights of Medication Administration

Any time you are asked to administer a medication, make sure you are adhering to the five rights of medication administration.

In addition, you must always accurately document any medication that you give in the patient's medical record.

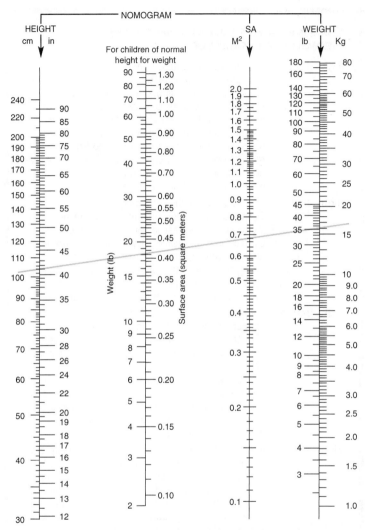

FIGURE 12–1. To calculate the body surface area (BSA), draw a line between the weight of a patient and the height of a patient. In the example shown, the BSA is 0.69.

THE FIVE RIGHTS FOR ADMINISTERING MEDICATION CORRECTLY

Right drug   Prepare the medication from the written order in the patient's medical record. In hospitals, drugs are prepared from transcribed medication orders. Check the label of the bottle or package containing the drug against the medication order to be sure they are the same. The label should be checked three times: (1) when the bottle is removed from the medication drawer or cabinet, (2) when the medication is removed from the bottle, and (3) when the medication is returned to storage.

Right dose   The drug is prescribed to achieve a specific effect. Giving too little medication may be ineffective; giving too much may cause harm to the patient. If a calculation is necessary, calculate the dose accurately before preparing the medication and work from your written calculation. If you have questions, ask another staff member to verify your calculation. Measure liquid medications accurately.

Right patient Always verify that medication is being given to the correct patient. To do this in an ambulatory care setting, take the patient's medical record with the medication to the patient. Ask the patient to state his or her name and verify it from the page of the medical record that contains the written medication order. In a hospital setting, the patient's name can be verified from the identification bracelet and checked against the written medication-administration record.

Right time   In the doctor's office, the time of day is usually less important than the interval between doses, as, for example, a series of hepatitis B immunizations or diptheria, pertussis, and tetanus (DPT) immunizations. Verify that the correct amount of time has passed since the last dose of the medication and refer any questions to the physician.

Right route   The medication must be given by the correct route to have the desired effect and, in the case of some injections, to prevent tissue injury. When giving injections, choose a needle length that will deposit the medication into the desired tissue based on the size of the patient and angle of administration. If you have questions, clarify the order with the physician.

Preparing and Administering Medication

Administering medication is one of the most important activities you will perform as a medical assistant. Always adhere to the following principles for safe preparation and administration of medication:

1. Never give medication without a valid order from a doctor or other licensed professional.
2. Check the expiration date and medication before preparing. Discard any discolored or expired medication.
3. Check the label three times to be sure you are preparing the correct medication. Check it when you remove the medication from storage, when you pour or draw up the medication, and when you return the medication bottle to storage.
4. Bring the prepared medication, the medical record, or a prepared-medication card and any other necessary supplies to the patient in one trip if possible so the patient is not left in an exam room alone with medication.
5. Identify the patient before giving any medication to be sure the correct patient is receiving the correct medication.
6. Always ask the patient (or the patient's caregiver if necessary) if the patient has any allergy before giving medication.
7. Administer medication by the route ordered by the practitioner.
8. Observe the patient taking oral medication; do not leave the patient to take medication alone.
9. Wear gloves if there is any possibility of coming into contact with body fluids.
10. When giving an injection, massage the injection site after administration to facilitate absorption. (The exceptions to this are injections of insulin or heparin, as well as intradermal injections.)
11. For an injection, select an appropriate site for the type, amount, and route of medication in order to avoid nerve, tissue, and/or blood vessel damage.
12. Always aspirate before injecting by the subcutaneous or intramuscular route to be sure the tip of the needle is not in a blood vessel. If blood enters the syringe, withdraw the needle and prepare a new injection for administration at another site.
13. Never break, recap, or bend a used needle.
14. Dispose of used needle and syringe in a rigid biohazard container (sharps container) as quickly as possible.

15. Never leave a biohazard container that contains used needles in the exam room unless it is attached to the wall and tamper proof.

16. Document all medication you give immediately after administration. Record the name of the medication, the dose as ordered, the route, and any untoward reactions that may have occurred.

ROUTES AND SITES FOR ADMINISTRATION OF PARENTERAL MEDICATION

Parenteral medication is administered by medical assistants by one of three routes. Some routes have multiple sites where medication may be administered. The three routes are:

- Subcutaneous
- Intramuscular
- Intradermal

Subcutaneous

Subcutaneous injections are given into the layer of fatty tissue below the skin. Proper sites for subcutaneous injections are those where there is a substantial layer of fatty tissue, such as the lateral aspect of the upper arm, about 3 inches above the elbow; the abdomen; the top of the leg; and the back, below the shoulder blades. Subcutaneous injections should be aspirated to make sure the needle is not in a blood vessel. After injection, massage the injection site to facilitate absorption and decrease discomfort (except for injections of heparin or insulin).

Figure 12–2 shows injection sites for subcutaneous injections.

Intramuscular Injections

Intramuscular injections are given directly into muscle tissue. Intramuscular injections are usually absorbed rapidly, but some oil-based preparations are long acting. These often contain the prefix *Depo-* in the name; a *depot* is a storage place. There are three preferred sites for an intramuscular injection in an adult:

- The deltoid injection site, in the upper arm, shown in Figure 12–3 (p. 160), is the most common site for intramuscular injections in the medical office.
- The dorsogluteal injection site, in the upper quadrant of the

Front   Back

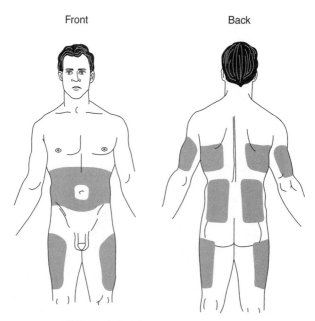

FIGURE 12–2. Subcutaneous injection sites.

buttock, shown in Figure 12–4 (p. 161), is the traditional site for deep intramuscular injections or injections that contain more fluid than 1 to 2 mL.

- The ventrogluteal injection site, on the side of the hip, shown in Figure 12–5 (p. 162), is relatively free of nerves. Although this site is more frequently used with hospitalized patients than in the ambulatory care setting, it is an excellent site for an intramuscular injection.

When giving an intramuscular injection, select the appropriate site, spread the skin with the thumb and forefinger, and administer the injection at a 90° angle.

Different sites can absorb different amounts of medication. The site should be chosen for safety and absorption of the particular amount and type of medication. If too much medication is absorbed into a small muscle, there may be tissue damage and/or poor absorption.

The preferred injection site for infants or toddlers is the vastus lateralis, on the outside of the upper leg, shown in Figure 12–6 (p. 163). This site is used because infants and toddlers have not yet

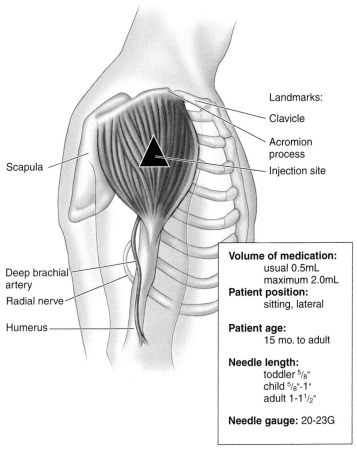

Landmarks:

Clavicle

Acromion process

Injection site

Scapula

Deep brachial artery

Radial nerve

Humerus

Volume of medication:
usual 0.5mL
maximum 2.0mL
Patient position:
sitting, lateral

Patient age:
15 mo. to adult

Needle length:
toddler ⁵/₈"
child ⁵/₈"-1"
adult 1-1¹/₂"

Needle gauge: 20-23G

FIGURE 12–3. The deltoid injection site.

developed the musculature of the back and buttock to absorb the fluid of the injection.

When a medication is extremely irritating to the subcutaneous tissue, the z-track method, illustrated in Figure 12–7 (p. 164), is used for injection to reduce the chance °F irritation. The dorsogluteal site is always used for a z-track injection. Before performing a z-track injection, make sure to change needles after medication has been drawn up and before it is injected in case some of the medication adheres to the outside of the needle.

To perform a z-track injection, with the fingers of your nondominant hand, pull the skin at the injection site to the left of its usual position about 2 to 3 inches. Hold the tissue to the side while you inject and aspirate. If no blood appears, slowly inject the medication. Then withdraw the needle swiftly, simultaneously releasing the tissue being held. Apply pressure to the site using a gauze pad and do not massage the site.

Intradermal

Intradermal injections are used for allergy testing and the Mantoux tuberculosis test (0.1 mL of purified protein derivative drawn up in a

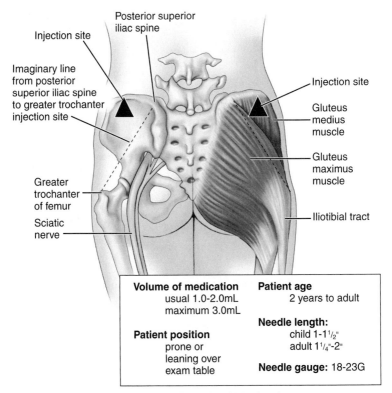

FIGURE 12–4. The dorsogluteal injection site.

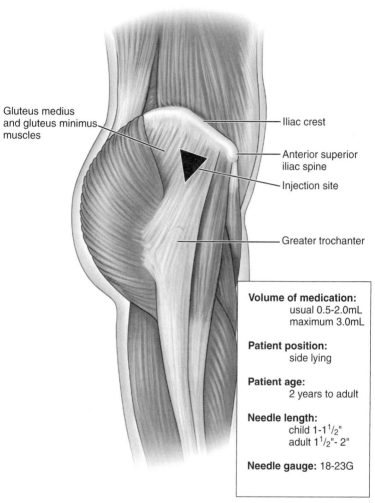

Gluteus medius
and gluteus minimus
muscles

Iliac crest

Anterior superior
iliac spine

Injection site

Greater trochanter

Volume of medication:
usual 0.5-2.0mL
maximum 3.0mL

Patient position:
side lying

Patient age:
2 years to adult

Needle length:
child 1-1$\frac{1}{2}$"
adult 1$\frac{1}{2}$"- 2"

Needle gauge: 18-23G

FIGURE 12–5. The ventrogluteal injection site.

tuberculin syringe). A 26 to 28 gauge (⅜- to ½-inch) needle is used for an intradermal injection.

Proper sites for an intradermal injection include the inner (anterior) forearm, the upper arm, the upper chest, or across the back. If giving a series of intradermal injections for allergy testing, the sites on the back allow several substances to be tested simultaneously.

When giving an intradermal injection using one of the sites shown in Figure 12–8 (p. 165), it is not necessary to aspirate the injection. Insert the needle between the layers of the skin at a 15° angle. Slowly inject the substance under the skin.

When the fluid is injected, it forces the epidermis to separate from

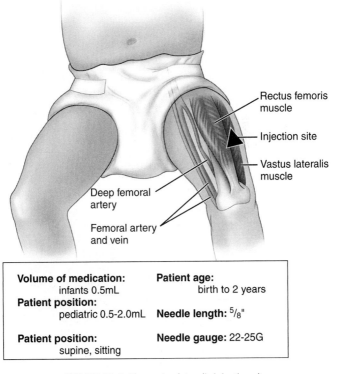

FIGURE 12–6. The vastus lateralis injection site.

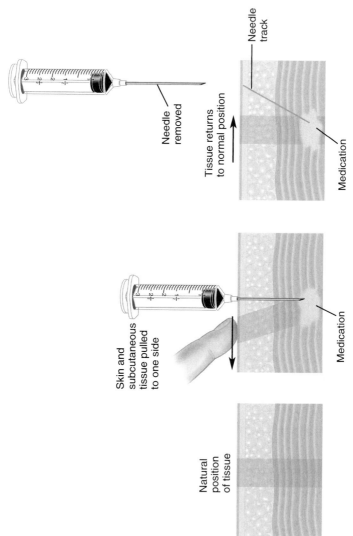

Natural
position
of tissue

Skin and
subcutaneous
tissue pulled
to one side

Medication

Tissue returns
to normal position

Needle
removed

Needle
track

Medication

FIGURE 12-7. Giving an injection using the z-track method.

Front   Back

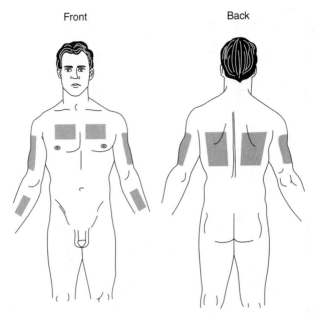

FIGURE 12–8. Intradermal injection sites.

the dermis. The raised area is called a wheal, or a bleb. If the needle penetrates too deeply, the wheal will not form. Remove the needle at the same angle at which you inserted it. There may be a small amount of capillary bleeding.

When performing a Mantoux test, ask the patient before the test if he or she has ever had a positive reaction to a test for tuberculosis. The test should not be performed on a patient who has had a positive reaction in the past because successive reactions tend to become more intense and are painful for the patient. A person who has been immunized for tuberculosis (a procedure that is not performed in the United States because it is believed to be ineffective, but that is performed in some other countries) should also not receive a Mantoux test because he or she will always have a positive reaction. The physician should be informed because a chest x-ray must be ordered in order to test for tuberculosis if a person is expected to have a positive reaction to a Mantoux test.

The Mantoux test is usually done on the forearm. The patient should be instructed to return in 48 to 72 hours so that you can read

TABLE 12-4
Controlled Substances

Schedule	Description	Legal Restrictions	Examples
Schedule I	No accepted medical use; high potential for addiction and/or abuse	May only be used in certain controlled research experiments	Heroin, marijuana, lysergic acid (LSD), mescaline, peyote
Schedule II	High potential for addiction and/or abuse; narcotics; stimulants such as cocaine and amphetamines; depressants in the barbiturate group	Can be prescribed only by MD who has received a license from the DEA (DEA number); requires a handwritten prescription with DEA number; prescription cannot be refilled; a special prescription form is used in many states.	Morphine, injectable codeine, secobarbital (Seconal), meperidine, methadone, methylphenidate (Ritalin); oxycodone (Percodan, Percocet)
Schedule III	Potential for dependence but lesser potential for abuse; combination drugs may contain small amounts of narcotics or amphetamine-like substances	Requires handwritten prescription; up to 5 refills in 6 months as written on the original prescription	Codeine in combination with non-narcotic drugs (e.g., acetaminophen with codeine); anabolic steroids, hydrocodone and butalbital compounds in combination with non-narcotic drugs
Schedule IV	Minor tranquilizers and sleep-inducing medications with less potential for abuse	Up to 5 refills in 6 months; prescription requires MD signature but refills may be authorized by telephone	Chlordiazepoxide (Librium), diazepam (Valium), phenobarbital, flurazepam (Dalmane), chloral hydrate, propoxyphene (Darvon)
Schedule V	Miscellaneous mixtures containing limited amounts of narcotic drugs; cough syrups containing codeine; less potential for abuse	Prescriptions and refills are the same as Schedule IV	Diphenoxylate (Lomotil); various cold and cough syrups such as brompheniramine and guaifenesin in preparations that contain codeine

the test. If there is a reaction, measure the area of induration (raised, hard, and reddened area) in millimeters, record it, and report it to the physician.

CONTROLLED SUBSTANCES

Table 12–4 summarizes information about controlled substances. Many offices avoid having controlled substances on the premises to decrease the likelihood of theft. If controlled substances are present, they must be stored in a cabinet with two locks (i.e., a locked cabinet within a locked cabinet.) They should be counted every day (or every shift if the facility is open around the clock) by two people who sign to validate that the count is correct. If it is necessary to waste a small amount of a controlled substance, two people should witness that it has been poured down the sink, and both should sign to validate this.

Chapter 13

Assisting with Surgery

INSTRUMENTS AND SUPPLIES COMMONLY USED FOR OFFICE SURGERY

Instruments

Various instruments and supplies may be necessary for office-based surgery. Surgical instruments are made of plastic, glass, or rubber. They are used for cutting, scraping, holding or grasping, pulling back (retracting), or suturing (stitching). They include a number of different types of forceps, scissors, scalpels and blades, retractors, probes and sounds, and curettes.

Among the instruments most frequently used for surgery are:

- Kelly hemostatic forceps (also called a hemostat or clamp), used to grasp bleeding blood vessels and also to clamp tubing (Fig. 13–1A)
- Needle holder (with shorter and thicker jaws than the Kelly hemostatic forceps), used to hold the needle during suturing (Fig. 13–1B)
- Tissue forceps, which have teeth to grasp tissue after the surgical incision has been made (Fig. 13–1C)
- Dressing forceps (also called thumb forceps), used to pick up sterile sponges or gauze squares (Fig. 13–1D)
- Operating scissors with sharp or blunt blades, used to cut tissue, for blunt dissection, or to cut suture material (Fig. 13–1E)
- Fine-point splinter forceps, used to remove foreign bodies from wounds (Fig. 13–1F)

Other instruments that may be used for sterile or nonsterile procedures include:

- Suture (stitch) scissors, used for removing sutures (Fig. 13–2A)
- Lister bandage scissors, used to cut dressings and tape (Fig. 13–2B)
- Sponge forceps, used to hold sponges during surgery and also used as sterile transfer forceps to move items on a sterile field (Fig. 13–2C)

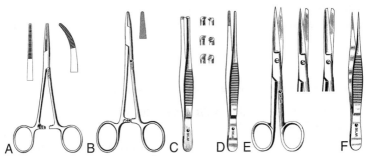

FIGURE 13–1. A, Kelly hemostatic forceps. B, Baumgartner needle holder. C, Tissue forceps. D, Dressing forceps. E, Operating scissors with three sets of cutting blades (sharp-sharp, sharp-blunt, and blunt-blunt). F, Fine-point splinter forceps. (Courtesy of Sklar Instruments, Westchester, Pennsylvania.)

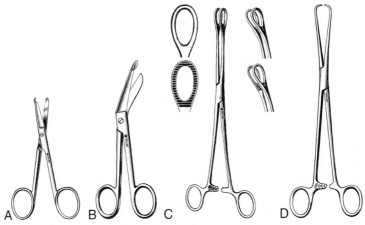

FIGURE 13–2. A, Spencer stitch scissors. B, Lister bandage scissors. C, Foerster sponge forceps. D, Tenaculum forceps. (Courtesy of Sklar Instruments, Westchester, Pennsylvania.)

- Tenaculum forceps, used to grasp the cervix during gynecologic procedures (Fig. 13–2D)

Supplies

In order to perform surgery or another sterile procedure, the physician needs sterile gauze squares (sponges), which come in sterile packages of two or can be added to surgical packs before sterilization in the office. Sterile wicking, a length of narrow sterile gauze, comes in a bottle and is used to pack deep wounds that must heal from inside out.

CARE OF INSTRUMENTS THAT MUST BE STERILIZED

1. Immediately after they are used, instruments should be soaked in a room-temperature, neutral pH solution to prevent blood and other biological material from drying. A plastic basin should be used to prevent instrument edges and tips from being damaged.
2. After the procedure is over, the medical assistant needs to clean and sterilize the equipment. To clean, always wear protective equipment (apron, mask, eye protection, and heavy-duty rubber gloves).
3. Carefully separate sharp instruments from other instruments that might have been soaking together. This reduces the likelihood of being cut by a sharp instrument every time you reach into the soak basin and reduces the likelihood that sharp instruments will be damaged. Also remove instruments that contain rubber (which can decompose if left in soaking solution too long) and plastic (which can discolor and lose its strength from soaking too long).
4. Wash each instrument thoroughly, checking to make sure it is in good working order. A soft bristle brush can be used to clean the ratchets, hinges, and serrated edges.
5. Dry each instrument thoroughly to avoid water spotting (even "stainless steel" will develop water stains). Separate instruments by the type of material used (stainless steel, chrome plate, and so on). Don't stack instruments on top of each other. Instruments with ratchets should be left with ratchets open.
6. Wrap instruments for sterilization with ratchets open. Place gauze squares to protect sharp blades or tips to prevent perforation of the wrap. Label and date all wrapped instruments and sterilize.

Draw the desired amount from the bottle using sterile forceps and cut with a sterile scissors.

Various solutions are used during sterile procedures, such as sterile water, sterile saline, liquid soap, and antiseptic solutions (e.g., povidone-iodine [Betadine]). Hydrogen peroxide is used to clean an incision before removing sutures. Do not touch the inside of the cap of a bottle containing solution used for sterile procedures.

Local anesthetic, such as lidocaine (Xylocaine), comes in various concentrations, with or without epinephrine. It is usually stored with other medications, and the bottle of anesthetic that the doctor wishes to use will be placed beside the sterile field for the medical assistant to hold when the doctor is ready to draw it up. A sterile syringe and needle is dropped onto the sterile field for this purpose.

Suture material, usually with an attached needle (swaged needle), comes with an outer package that can be peeled open to drop the sterile inner package on the sterile field. The medical assistant should be sure to open the correct type and size of suture material and needle desired by the physician.

Sterile drapes and towels, usually disposable, of various types may be used to create a sterile field and/or frame the surgical site. A package containing sterile towels should also be opened for drying the hands after a surgical aseptic handwashing.

PROCEDURE FOR SURGICAL ASEPTIC HANDWASHING

1. Remove all jewelry and store in safe, secure place.
2. Open package of sterile towels.
3. Using foot controls, regulate water to a comfortably warm temperature and rinse hands and forearms, holding them upright at or above waist level.
4. Clean under and around nails with brush or wooden orange stick. Apply adequate soap and scrub one hand and forearm and then the other, fingertips up, with a surgical scrub brush, using friction, for at least 3 minutes. Lather and scrub without touching faucet or sink.
5. Discard brush. Rinse hands and forearms thoroughly, holding hands and arms up.

(continued)

**PROCEDURE FOR SURGICAL ASEPTIC
HANDWASHING** *Continued*

6. If using foot or elbow controls, turn off water; otherwise, leave water running for someone else to turn off. Hold hands above waist.

7. Pick up the sterile towel without touching the package and dry one hand from hand to arm. Use a new towel for the second arm. Drop each towel (rather than putting it down) after use to avoid contaminating hands.

8. Hold hands up and in front of your body until you can apply sterile gloves.

PROCEDURE FOR APPLYING STERILE GLOVES

1. Remove all jewelry, store in safe secure place, and perform a surgical aseptic handwash.

2. Place package of sterile gloves on flat surface at waist level.

3. Open package, being careful not to touch sterile inner packet because your hands are never sterile.

4. Grasp the edge of the inner packet and pull the paper open to expose both sterile gloves inside, touching only the edges of the package to keep the area sterile.

5. With the fingers and thumb of your dominant hand, pick up the glove for the other hand by grasping the inside of the glove. Pull the glove on without touching the outside.

6. With gloved hand, pick up the second glove by placing gloved fingers between the folded cuff and the fingers of the second glove (Fig. 13–3).

7. Slip the second hand into the glove, making sure not to let the gloved hand touch the skin of the nongloved hand.

8. Once hands are in gloves, hold them above the waist. You may adjust the fingers with the other hand, but do not touch anything that is not sterile.

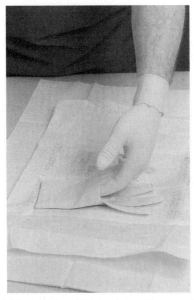

FIGURE 13–3. The correct position to pick up the second sterile glove.

Setting Up a Sterile Field

The sterile field is the area on which sterile instruments and supplies can be prepared so they stay sterile before and during a procedure. A sterile field can be formed from a square or rectangular cloth or paper. The sterile field is set up either on a countertop or on a Mayo stand. You may use either instruments sterilized in an autoclave or disposable surgical packs, prepackaged with disposable instruments and supplies necessary to perform a single procedure.

The following eight rules should be followed at all times:

1. Use only sterile objects to touch other sterile objects. Once a sterile object has been touched with an object that is not sterile, the formerly sterile object is no longer sterile.
2. Only areas in your direct line of vision are sterile. If you can't see it, you must assume it is not sterile. Always keep the sterile field in your vision. If you must leave the area, back away from the sterile field so you do not contaminate it by accident.
3. Only the area above waist level is sterile. The draping around the sterile field that falls below the table level is not sterile. If you lower

your hands below waist level, they are no longer sterile. Anything that falls to the floor, obviously, is no longer sterile. In addition, the outside 1 inch of the sterile field on all sides is to be considered nonsterile; sterile items should always be placed in the middle of the sterile field.

4. Avoid passing nonsterile objects over the sterile field. In fact, don't reach over the sterile field at all, if possible. Once used, do not return sterile instruments, sponges, or supplies to the sterile field.

5. When pouring sterile liquids, avoid splashing. The area below the field is not sterile, and if the field becomes wet, it can wick up harmful microorganisms. Don't let the edge of a bottle touch the sterile item (bowl or basin) that you are pouring onto.

6. Don't sneeze, cough, or talk above the sterile field. Microorganisms from the respiratory system contaminate the sterile field and the objects on it.

7. Cover the sterile field with a sterile towel if it will not be under direct observation by anyone for even a moment.

8. When a physician puts on a sterile gown before the procedure, you can assist by tying it in back. The front of the gown above the waist

---

PROCEDURE FOR PREPARING A STERILE FIELD

1. Wash hands.

2. Place package with sterile drape on a flat surface near where sterile field will be set up and open package without touching the drape.

3. Step away from surface as you pick up drape, allowing it to unfold without touching anything, then lay the drape over the Mayo stand or part of counter where the sterile field will be located.

4. Add sterile items to the sterile field.

5. Open plastic and/or paper peel packs carefully and flip the inner contents onto the field without touching them or the sterile field.

6. To pour solutions, open the bottle and place the lid inside, facing up beside the field. Pour a small amount of solution into the sink, then hold the bottle about 4 inches above a sterile container and pour the desired amount of solution without touching the sterile container.

7. Put on sterile gloves or use a sterile sponge forceps to touch or adjust items on the sterile field.

and the lower half of the front sleeves are the parts of the gown that are considered sterile.

Preparing the Skin

The area of skin where the surgical incision will be made needs to be as free of bacterial and other pathogens as possible. It is never possible to totally sterilize the skin, but it is possible to keep almost all harmful organisms away from the surgical site.

Assisting with Minor Surgery

Once a sterile field has been established and the surgical equipment and supplies are laid out on the sterile field, and once the patient is prepped and draped, surgery can begin. Depending on the complexity of the procedure and time it will take, you will have different responsibilities.

Nonsterile Assistant

If you are not sterile, you may not touch any of the sterile items on the field. However, you can:

- Tie the back of the surgeon's sterile gown
- Get supplies and add them to the sterile field
- Reassure the patient
- Adjust the light for the doctor
- Adjust the doctor's mask, face shield, and/or protective glasses and wipe sweat from the doctor's forehead as necessary
- Clean and hold a bottle of local antiseptic for the physician to insert a sterile needle and draw up solution
- Hold a container to receive any specimen for biopsy

Sterile Assistant

For simple procedures, you may wear only sterile gloves. For more complex procedures, you may also wear a mask, hat, sterile gown, and sterile gloves. If you are sterile, you may:

- Hand instruments to the doctor
- Hold a retractor
- Suction or sponge blood from the surgical site, using a sterile tip or sterile gauze sponges.

PROCEDURE FOR PREPARING THE SKIN FOR A STERILE PROCEDURE

1. Wash hands and assemble equipment.
2. Identify and greet the patient, explain the procedure, and check both the patient's chart and verbally with the patient for any allergies to iodine or shellfish.
3. Open sterile basin(s) and pour solution(s). Open razor for surgical prep.
4. Put on sterile gloves.
5. Apply antiseptic soap with gauze sponge, beginning at the site where the incision will be made and moving outward. Use a circular motion. Scrub for 2 to 5 minutes, but don't abrade the skin.
6. Hold skin taut and shave hair in the direction of hair growth if there is hair. Rinse and wash skin a second time after shaving.
7. Rinse with sterile solution as requested by the doctor. Dry with gauze sponges or sterile towel.
8. Remove and discard soiled sterile gloves and soiled/wet underpad, and replace underpad under surgical site. Discard razor in a sharps container. Discard solutions and supplies in the appropriate areas.
9. If instructed by the physician, put on new sterile gloves and apply povidone–iodine solution to the area cleaned using prepackaged swabs or povidone–iodine solution in a sterile bowl and sterile swabs. Apply in a circular motion, moving outward from the proposed incision site. Allow to air dry and cover with a sterile towel if the physician is not ready to proceed.

Procedure Cards

When setting up for a surgical procedure, it is helpful to use a surgical-procedure card that identifies the specifics of the procedure and the doctor's preferences. An example of a general card is shown in Figure 13–4. If you are assigned to assist with an unfamiliar procedure, you may want to look up the procedure in the office procedure manual and create your own card.

Procedure Card for Minor Surgery

Supplies and Equipment:

For the doctor: Open sterile gown, sterile gloves, sterile towel. The doctor will put on surgical cap, shoe covers and mask before washing hands.

Sterile Pack: Assemble needed equipment such as surgical scissors, scalpel, hemostats, sterile bowls, etc.

Other Supplies: Betadine swab sticks, Xylocaine 1%, 3 ml syringe with 25G 5/8" needle attached, sterile 0.9% saline solution, Betadine solution, alcohol wipes, 1 inch cloth tape, fenestrated drape, bottle containing Formalin for specimens (if needed), sterile swabs for culture, sterile sponge forceps.

Patient position: Position the patient as indicated for the specific procedure.

Prepare sterile field: Open sterile pack on Mayo stand. Use sterile sponge forceps to arrange. Pour solutions into sterile bowls if needed. Add 3 mL syringe with needle for local anesthetic. Add suture material if needed. Add any other instruments requested by the physician if not included in the sterile pack.

FIGURE 13–4. A surgical-procedure card that identifies the preferences of the doctor performing the surgery is useful to prepare supplies and equipment.

Figure continued on following page

Procedure Card for Minor Surgery

Assist the doctor • Tie gown, adjust mask if needed.

• Clean stopper and hold Xylocaine bottle upside down with label facing the doctor who will draw up the local anesthetic.

• Open Betadine swabsticks without touching ends of swabs and hold for the doctor to remove.

• Open package holding fenestrated drape and hold for the doctor to remove.

• If a specimen is to be sent to the lab, open bottle containing Formalin for the doctor to add specimen or hold culture transport medium for the doctor to insert swab for culture.

FIGURE 13–4 *Continued.*

Removing Sutures or Staples

Sutures and/or staples used to hold an incision are often removed in the medical office, even if the surgery itself was done in the emergency room or in an operating room. The physician should always assess the incision to be sure that healing has occurred, but you will set up for the procedure and may be instructed by the physician to remove the staples or sutures. Wear gloves to remove any dressings so the physician can see the incision, if needed. Discard soiled dressings in a biohazard waste container. If the incision contains crusts, clean with a sterile swab using hydrogen peroxide or other solution as directed by the physician.

To remove staples, wear gloves and use a sterile staple remover (often disposable). Slide the staple remover carefully under each staple to be removed. Press the handles together so the ends slide out of the skin. Place each staple on a gauze square as it is removed. Instruct the patient how to care for the incision and apply a light dressing if the patient wants to protect the incision from pressure. Always compare the number of staples removed to the number inserted, if possible, and document the number of staples removed and the appearance of the incision.

To remove sutures, use sterile stitch scissors (see Fig. 13–2A, p. 169) and sterile dressing forceps (see Fig. 13–1D, p. 169). These often come in a disposable suture-removal kit. Prepare the patient in the same way as described for removing staples. When the incision has been cleaned, put on gloves. Use the forceps to grasp one of the ends of the suture, near the knot. Apply tension, slide the curved part of the scissors under the suture, and cut. Pull each suture out with the forceps and lay it on a clean gauze square for easy counting. As with staples, the appearance of the incision and number of sutures removed should be documented.

Transdisciplinary Competencies

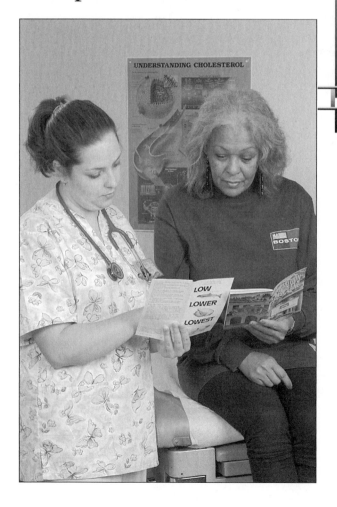

Chapter 14

Facilitating Communication

VERBAL AND NONVERBAL COMMUNICATION

You communicate with others not only by what you say and how you say it but also through a set of nonverbal cues, including your body language, your tone of voice, how you enter a room, the facial expressions you use, and the gestures you make while speaking.

Explicit use of body language can help you present yourself as a professional (e.g., good posture, purposeful strides). Body language can also help you project empathy with your patients (e.g., sitting close but not too close, making eye contact, nodding as the patient relates his or her purpose for the visit).

You should also be mindful of the nonverbal messages sent by others. Some patients want a sense of intimacy, while others wish to maintain a certain distance. Try not to overwhelm others with your natural nonverbal communications; learn to match your nonverbal behavior to cues being presented by others.

COMMUNICATION TECHNIQUES THAT DEMONSTRATE ACTIVE LISTENING

Active listening is perhaps the most important communication skill a medical assistant can learn. In the current health care system, there is increasing pressure for doctors and other licensed professionals to see more and more patients each day. As a medical assistant, you may be able to give patients more of the "hand holding" they wish for and need to meet their health care needs.

Active listening means paying attention with your entire mind to what is being said, being "in the moment" with the other party in the conversation. When engaged in a conversation with a patient, don't be thinking of other things; focus all of your attention on the other person. Let the other person carry the conversation, and use your skills to gently steer it and keep it on track, rather than managing the conversation rigorously.

The "real" reason for a patient visit may come out more in the conversation around the history of the present illness than it does in objective signs of illness. When listening:

- Listen for feelings.
- Be observant.
- Be patient and listen completely.

Table 14–1 describes in more detail some techniques for active listening.

TABLE 14–1
Communication Techniques That Demonstrate Active Listening

Technique	Description	Example
Using open-ended questions	Asking questions that do not expect a particular answer, especially a *yes* or *no* answer	Medical assistant: "What's been going on lately?" "Tell me about your stomach pain."
Repeating or rephrasing	Saying the same thing as the patient either as a statement or a question to encourage agreement, disagreement, or clarification	Patient: "It feels like someone is stabbing me in the side." Medical assistant: "Like a knife in your side . . . "
Translating into feelings	Translating the patient's message into a verbal expression of emotion	Patient: "All the doctor visits, the medication, the pain—it's really too much." Medical assistant: "You sound like you feel overwhelmed."
Reflecting	Turning a question or statement around to reflect back to the patient; this gives the patient confidence to continue	Patient: "Would you have this surgery if you were me?" Medical assistant: "What do you think about having the surgery?"

TABLE 14–1 Communication Techniques That Demonstrate Active Listening *Continued*		
Technique	*Description*	*Example*
Paraphrasing and summarizing	Paraphrasing puts the patient's statement into the medical assistant's own words; summarizing restates the meaning but may leave out some of the details; the purposes are to validate that the medical assistant has understood and encourage clarification	Medical assistant: "So for the past week, the pain has been getting steadily more intense and more frequent, and since this morning it hasn't let up at all."
Providing silence	Simply waiting for the patient to continue; allows the patient to choose whether to continue or choose a new topic	(Silence)
Verbalizing the implied	Saying what the patient seems to mean but has not expressed	Patient: "Usually I don't mind coming to see Dr. Hughes." Medical assistant: "But you didn't want to come today . . . "
Asking for clarification	Asking for more detail or a clearer statement; lets the patient know that the medical assistant has not understood and may show the patient how to make the message clearer	Medical assistant: "It's not clear to me how often you have been taking this medication. Do you take it before every meal, or just when you are at home?"

BLOCKS TO COMMUNICATION

Blocks to effective communication can occur. The way you phrase a question or a response may be interpreted by the patient in such a way that he or she "turns off" the rest of the conversation.

Table 14–2 (p. 186) describes some of the more common communication blocks you should try to avoid.

TABLE 14–2
Blocks to Effective Communication

Type of Communication	Description	Example
Offering false reassurance	Telling the patient that everything will be all right; implies that the patient should not feel anxiety or concern; especially inappropriate when the medical assistant does not know what will happen	Medical assistant: "Don't worry, your husband will come through this with flying colors."
Disapproving, blaming	Making a negative value judgment about the patient's thinking or behavior; by implying or stating that a patient is responsible for his or her health problem, the medical assistant encourages the patient to defend against attack rather than establishing trust	Medical assistant: "You shouldn't be smoking anyway. No wonder you have trouble breathing."
Challenging	Insisting that the patient prove a statement or belief	Medical assistant: "Just show me something in writing that says people should never take a bath."
Defending	Protecting oneself or someone else from criticism, which implies that the patient does not have a right to have a different opinion	Medical assistant: "Dr. Lawler's patients never have to wait very long."
Asking for explanations of feelings or behavior	Because patients often don't know why they feel or act as they do, asking *why* may be frustrating and intrusive	Medical assistant: "Why don't you stick to your diet?"; "Why are you angry?"
Belittling or negating feelings	Acting as if feelings are less intense than they are or not even present; this implies that the patient's feelings are not real or not justified	Medical assistant: "You are really making a big deal out of a little cut."

TABLE 14–2 Blocks to Effective Communication *Continued*		
Type of Communication	**Description**	**Example**
Changing the subject	By not responding to a statement, especially if it expresses feelings, the medical assistant implies that the patient's feelings are inappropriate or can't be accepted	Patient: "Sometimes I am so down that I can't get out of bed." Medical assistant: "Would you just sit over here so I can take your temperature."
Stereotyping	Minimizing a person's unique experience by reducing people to generalized categories	Medical assistant: "You are just feeling upset because you are pregnant."

ADAPTING COMMUNICATION FOR PATIENTS WITH SPECIAL NEEDS

A number of patients in the medical office may have special needs relative to communication. These are sometimes referred to as barriers to communication. The five most common special circumstances are:

- Impaired level of understanding
- Impaired sensation caused by illness or disease
- Strong emotion
- Language (i.e., non–native-English speakers)
- Cultural differences

Impaired Understanding

In the case of an individual with an impaired level of understanding, it is important to simplify communications. Individuals with impaired understanding may be children, mentally retarded patients, or elderly patients experiencing some confusion or some level of dementia. To communicate with a patient whose level of understanding is impaired:

- Use short sentences.
- Use simple words.
- Maintain strong eye contact.
- Speak slowly, in a clear voice with normal volume.

- Express concern and empathy.
- Repeat what you say until understood, calmly and slowly.
- Ask the patient to repeat what you have said to be sure that he or she has understood.

Impaired Sensation

A patient with impaired eyesight or impaired hearing needs extra attention in the medical office. Both types of patients require extra care to move around the office and the examination room as well.

For a sight-impaired patient, you can either let the individual take your arm or use his or her cane to navigate the corridors. In the exam room, you should try to orient the person using a clock face as the reference (e.g., "Mr. Casey, the exam table is five steps from your chair, at about two o'clock.").

A hearing-impaired patient may need a gentle touch on the arm to get his or her attention. You should speak slowly, in a normal tone and volume, without overly broad facial gestures. Ask the patient if he or she reads lips or uses sign language or finger spelling. Be sure to supply written instructions for any test or procedure.

Emotions

Patients who are ill often display anxiety, fear, anger, or other strong emotions. This can temporarily impair their ability to both send and receive effective communication cues.

Getting informed consent from an emotionally impaired patient can be difficult. A person in a highly charged emotional state cannot legally sign a consent form. If you cannot help the individual return to a more neutral emotional state, any procedure requiring informed consent must be delayed.

Remember that patients experiencing strong emotions may say things that you should not take personally. Try to identify and help the patient verbalize the emotion rather than becoming defensive and arguing about the content of a patient's message. If the patient begins the interaction with a statement like, "Obviously my time is not important to anyone in this office," it is more effective to respond with a statement like, "You sound upset," than "We are working to see patients as fast as we can."

Language Barriers

The best way to work around language differences is with translation assistance, unless you are fluent in the patient's native language. Translators can be office staff, community volunteers, or family members. When making an appointment for a non–English-speaking patient, find out if a family member will be present to translate.

When using a translator to converse with a patient:

- Speak to the patient, not the translator.
- Speak slowly and carefully.
- Use short sentences and simple terms.
- Use gestures to reinforce your comments.

When using an interpreter, instruct him or her to translate the meaning of whoever is speaking, but focus your attention on the person with whom you are trying to communicate so that nonverbal communication can occur.

Appendix A contains some common words and phrases in Spanish. If the practice you are working in has a significant percentage of patients who speak a different foreign language, ask a native speaker to help you prepare a similar set of phrases in that language.

Cultural Differences

Try whenever possible to use a staff member or volunteer to translate. The use of a family member as translator often not only puts that person in the middle of the conversation but also forces that person to participate in any instructions you may give. This can put a strain on family relationships, especially when following medical instructions requires behavior changes that affect others in the patient's family.

This is especially true around issues of diet for weight and blood pressure control. Every culture has its comfort foods, and trying to get someone to change cooking and eating habits often requires the cooperation and support of others in the family.

Learn about cultural traditions of any significant patient group in your medical practice, and respect other cultural traditions.

Chapter 15

Legal Concepts

CONFIDENTIALITY

Information about a patient learned in the course of treatment is confidential. In order for that information to be shared with others who are not involved in direct care (i.e., other doctors to whom your office refers the patient, the doctor who referred the patient to your office, insurance providers, and so on), the patient must provide written consent.

- Never release any information to family, friends, or others who call except to the parents of children who are patients.
- Never gossip about patients. If it is necessary to discuss a patient with another staff member, do so in a private place.

Inappropriate release of information about a patient is an invasion of privacy. Every medical office has forms that patients must sign in order to provide consent for the sharing of medical information with others who need to know.

The one general exception about patient privacy is in the area of mandated public health or other reports. Certain diseases must be reported to the local board of health, suspected abuse must be reported to the proper state authorities, births and deaths must be reported, and injuries that may be the result of a crime must be reported to the local police department.

INFORMED CONSENT

Before performing any invasive procedure on a patient, the patient must give informed consent. A patient has the legal right to know and completely understand what will be done to or for him or her.

Before any procedure, the patient must be given a thorough explanation and reason for performing the procedure. For simple procedures, such as an injection, verbal consent is sufficient. For more extensive procedures, such as minor surgery or endoscopy, the patient should sign a written consent form, which states that the procedure has been explained to the patient and that the patient understands the nature of and reason for the procedure. Written consent is also required for HIV testing. Some offices are now asking parents to provide written consent for immunizations for their children.

The person performing the procedure is responsible for explaining it to the patient. In the medical office, as a medical assistant, you will often be the person who obtains written consent from the patient and witnesses the form. The form must be signed before any medication is administered that can alter the patient's mood or thinking process. If the patient does not appear to understand or still has questions about the procedure, be sure that the doctor or other provider speaks with the patient before obtaining the signature. Avoid making any promises about the outcome of the procedure while obtaining written consent. If the patient appears to be very concerned, refer him or her to the person who will perform the procedure.

LEGAL RESTRICTIONS

There are four general legal restrictions you should consider as a medical assistant:

1. A medical assistant cannot perform activities that are part of the practice of medicine.
   - Don't use diagnostic terms when documenting in the medical record.
   - Be sure that a doctor authorizes all prescription refills before contacting a pharmacy.
   - Don't instruct the patient to take medication unless there are written guidelines in your office that cover the patient's particular circumstances (e.g., a guideline that states that parents should give acetaminophen to a child with a fever higher than 101°F).
2. Don't administer medications unless it is legal for you to do so in

your state. Be sure that a doctor is present in the office if you do administer medication.

3. Don't perform a procedure for which you have not been trained. If you do so, you may be held to the standard of care of the licensed professional who usually performs such a procedure.

4. Abide by all laws of the state where you are working. If you work in a state other than the one in which you were trained, be sure you are thoroughly familiar with that state's laws as they pertain to medical assistants. For instance:

   • In some states, medical assistants may not administer medications.

   • In some states, medical assistants may not take x-rays or perform other specific procedures or diagnostic tests.

NEGLIGENCE/MALPRACTICE

Negligence is the failure to act or refrain from acting as a reasonable person would in any given circumstance.

Negligence within the practice of a profession is called malpractice. A professional is always held to the highest standard of that profession. So, in the professional context, a practitioner is required to act not merely as a reasonable person, but rather as a professional.

To avoid lawsuits for malpractice, a health care professional must be sure he or she is acting within the limits of his or her profession, and must act in a given situation as a reasonable and prudent professional would. Most office malpractice-insurance policies cover medical assistants as well as doctors and nurses; if your office's insurance coverage does not cover you, you can obtain professional liability/malpractice insurance through the American Association of Medical Assistants.

The accompanying box discusses measures you can take to avoid malpractice actions against yourself and others in the medical office.

RISK MANAGEMENT

Risk management is a term used to describe the measures taken and activities performed in a medical office that reduce physical risk to patients, staff, and visitors, and also the measures taken and activities performed to reduce the likelihood of a malpractice action being taken against a member of the office staff. Usually, the office manager is responsible for overseeing the risk-management effort.

MEASURES TO PREVENT MALPRACTICE

The best way to protect against lawsuits for malpractice is to use the proper procedures to prevent mistakes:

- Make sure all equipment is in good working order and that you have been properly trained to use it.
- Make sure you know how to do procedures, and review them in the procedure manual before performing them if you have any doubts.
- Be sure patients understand the nature of procedures and surgery, and always obtain written consent for surgery and other invasive procedures.
- Always document accurately and completely. Report any problems promptly, and document your report.
- Protect patients from injury by using equipment correctly. Assist patients to transfer to and from wheelchairs.
- Don't leave patients alone if there is any question of their balance or mental status. Don't ever leave children unattended in an exam room or the waiting room.
- Use care to identify any patient specimens. Label all specimens correctly. Log and track all results, and be sure patients are notified if lab results are abnormal.
- Never leave a patient unattended with hot packs or where there is hot water or hot pipes.
- Clean liquid spills promptly and put up signs if floors are wet.
- Don't make promises about the outcome of a procedure or surgery.
- Keep current on procedures and equipment, and get training as necessary.
- Notify a doctor of any patient complaints or requests for patient records.
- Always follow up with patients who have had surgical procedures.

Risk management involves a process of assessing risks and putting in place policies and procedures that minimize risk. Risk in a medical office comes in many forms:

- Physical risk of injury or illness
- Malpractice liability risk
- Business risk (e.g., failure to diligently collect bills)

Whenever a new policy is adopted or a new procedure is put in place to reduce risk, every employee covered by the policy or procedure must be educated about it. Policy and procedure manuals, once developed, must be accessible to all employees.

Incident Reports

Whenever something happens in the office for which the office could be considered legally liable, an incident report should be filled out. Find out where to obtain a form and how to complete it. The incident report is initiated by the staff member who was involved in the incident or most closely witnessed the incident. Incident reports should be filled out when:

- Anyone (employee, patient, or visitor) falls in the office
- There is a medication error
- Blood is drawn from the wrong patient
- The number of surgical instruments counted after a procedure does not match the number counted before the procedure
- An employee has a needle-stick injury

Information that needs to be included on an incident report is:

- Name, address, telephone number, date of birth, and gender of injured person
- Time of day, day, date, and exact location in the office where the incident occurred
- A brief narrative of the incident
- Any diagnostic procedures performed to assess the injury and/or any treatments provided for the injury
- Names, addresses, and phone numbers of any witnesses
- Signature and date of the person making the report

Chapter 16

Patient Instruction

People learn in a holistic manner. This means that they respond to all of the various stimuli in any given situation, not merely to what is said or written. When learning, a person internalizes new information, ideas, emotions, and behaviors. Providing information is not enough; a patient educator must stimulate the learner.

THE TEACHING PROCESS

There are six steps in the teaching process:

1. Identify a need for teaching.
2. Assess the learner.
3. Plan activities to meet learning needs.
4. Implement teaching.
5. Evaluate effectiveness of teaching and learning.
6. Document learning outcomes.

Identify Need

Identification of a teaching need often comes from something the patient says or does that suggests he or she does not understand the next step in a process. You may be able to prompt the patient to admit not knowing by asking some simple but probing questions.

When a patient is newly diagnosed with a chronic disease, you can assume that the individual needs education about the condition, daily care of the condition, and the medical regimen for treating the condition. The three most common chronic illnesses you will need to educate patients about are:

- Asthma (especially in children)

- Diabetes
- Heart disease

Assess Learner

Before planning and implementing education, you must assess not only what the patient knows about the subject but also how motivated the patient is to learn, what particular learning skills the patient has, and what barriers might inhibit learning.

After conducting this assessment, you can plan an education program using tools that work well with the patient's strong skills (e.g., learning by doing, learning from pictures) while downplaying the patient's weaker learning skills (e.g., low reading comprehension).

Plan Activities

A teaching plan can be as simple as deciding to give a particular patient a two-sentence response to a question. Or it can be as complex as an outline for a multisession education plan. Identify written materials, such as brochures or pamphlets, that you can give the patient to reinforce teaching. Each office usually keeps a variety of materials that have been approved by the physicians.

When planning teaching, you need to:

- Identify learning goals (desired outcomes).
- Identify actions to be taken to meet those goals (teaching strategies).
- Identify particular tools to use with each strategy.

Implement Teaching

Teaching sessions are most effective when they are short and focus on a discreet set of activities or tasks. Review the material from the last session before going on to new material. When a patient needs to learn how to perform a particular procedure, schedule several sessions for the patient to practice. Provide coaching, assistance, and encouragement.

Use standardized materials whenever possible. This both reduces the amount of lesson development you need to do and ensures consistency and accuracy of the material presented. However, you should personalize the delivery of even standard material for each individual patient.

Evaluate Effectiveness

Goals and objectives for patient education need to be measurable so they can be evaluated. In more complex learning situations, each discreet objective should be evaluated individually in order to determine that the patient has mastered them all and thus mastered the entire teaching goal.

Document Outcomes

After each session, document the teaching done and identify what the patient said or did to demonstrate that he or she understands the material presented.

ADAPTING TO LEARNER NEEDS

As people develop from young children to adults to elders, their learning style often changes. Table 16–1 (p. 198) describes in detail the various ways of learning most common to people at different stages of development and the most effective teaching methods for individuals at these stages.

Sometimes you will need to adapt teaching for a specific learner. Factors that influence how you present the material include:

- Educational level
- Cultural factors
- Physical or mental impairment
- Language

Education

An individual's level of education affects the type of written information you can use. While highly educated people may wish detailed, written material, those with less formal education may need written material to be short and written in simple language, with a lot of illustrations to reinforce the message.

Culture

Culture often has an impact on individual lifestyle. Sometimes you will need to take cultural background into account when teaching patients. This is especially true in areas of diet and nutrition.

TABLE 16–1
Teaching and Learning at Different Stages of Development

Ways of Learning	Effective Teaching Methods
Infant	
Uses senses to explore environment	Help the infant to learn to trust his or her environment by holding securely, speaking softly, allowing time for visual and tactile exploration.
Learns to trust when held securely, changes introduced slowly, shown love and acceptance	
Toddler	
Learns to use language to communicate but still tends to express feelings through behavior	Use simple words, brief explanations. Use play to teach a procedure. Allow for imitation and play. Use praise to reinforce desired behavior.
Uses play to explore environment and imitation to learn new behavior	
Preschooler	
Still learning to use language correctly	Use role-playing, imitation, and play to teach.
Still tends to express feelings through actions rather than words	Use short sentences but reinforce with demonstration.
Asks questions to learn about environment	Encourage questions.
School-Aged Child	
Child learns to think about information abstractly and can memorize facts, safety rules, and procedures. Judgment improves.	Discussion can be reinforced by pamphlets, videos, and other visual aids, but level of language must not be too complex.
Learns from observation, discussion, reading, and experimentation.	Allow time for questions.
	Evaluate learning by having child summarize information or demonstrate skills.
Adolescent	
Can analyze, compare, make decisions, and solve abstract problems	Demonstrate problem-solving skills. Provide privacy and autonomy.
Emotionally challenged to adapt to body-image changes and manage intense feelings; wants to be responsible for self, but judgment may need development	Help to learn about feelings; demonstrate acceptance of intense feelings. Encourage responsible decision-making about health issues.

TABLE 16–1
Teaching and Learning at Different Stages of Development *Continued*

Ways of Learning	*Effective Teaching Methods*
Young and Middle-Aged Adult	
Has reached full cognitive development but may be overwhelmed by family, occupational, and social responsibilities	Allow participation in setting goals and determining appropriate learning activities.
Older Adult	
May have decreased vision, hearing, mobility, and strength; ability to think, remember, and control emotions may be decreased as well; usually needs longer time to respond and more repetition to remember	Treat with dignity, but use simpler language and louder and slower speech if necessary and allow time to respond. Teach in short sessions and observe for signs of fatigue, such as irritability or failure to pay attention.

Food plays a large role in some cultures, and dietary changes may have a profound effect not only on the individual's eating habits but also on the entire family's eating habits; even on the family dynamics within the household.

Impairment

Physical impairment not only affects how patient education is conducted, but in many instances necessitates education about how to adapt to those impairments.

This is true not only regarding assistive devices for ambulation (discussed later) but also in other ways. For instance, you may need to work with a patient with failing memory about how to keep track of pills using a weekly pill container.

Language

Patient education materials should be written in whatever languages are frequently spoken by patients in your office (within reason).

It is best if verbal instruction is given by an educator speaking in the patient's native language if possible, rather than through a translator.

COMMON INSTRUCTION TOPICS

Ambulatory Aids

Whenever an assistive device is to be used, the patient and a family member should be taught how to use the device safely and effectively.

A cane is the least cumbersome assistive device. Canes can be aluminum (adjustable) or wood. Whether a single-footed cane or a quad cane is to be used:

- The cane should be sized by making sure the top of the cane is even with the patient's hip.
- The cane should be held in the hand opposite the affected leg.
- The elbow should be bent 20° to 30°.
- The affected leg should advance 12 to 18 inches, and then the unaffected leg should be brought forward, slightly ahead of the cane.

Crutches have hand grips and are generally used in pairs. They can be made of aluminum or wood, and all are adjustable for height. There are three types of crutches:

- Axillary crutches, with rests that fit under the axilla
- Forearm (Canadian, Lofstrand) crutches, which are held in the hand and have a metal cuff that fits around the forearm
- Platform crutches, which have a shelflike device and straps to support the forearm

Crutches can be used in several different ways, depending on how much weight the affected leg or legs can support. There are five basic crutch gaits, as illustrated in Figure 16–1:

- Two-point gait, in which each leg is moved along with the opposite crutch, used when both legs need some support
- Three-point gait, in which both crutches are moved along with the affected leg, used for either a non–weight-bearing or partial weight-bearing affected leg
- Four-point gait, in which each crutch and each leg is moved independently, used for partial weight bearing on both legs, when both need support
- Swing-to gait, in which both crutches are moved forward, then both legs are swung up to a position even with the crutches

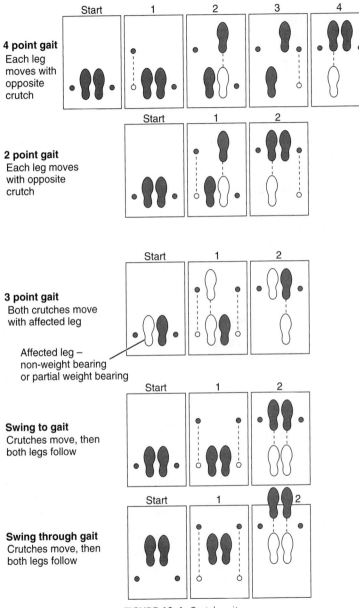

4 point gait
Each leg moves with opposite crutch

2 point gait
Each leg moves with opposite crutch

3 point gait
Both crutches move with affected leg

Affected leg – non-weight bearing or partial weight bearing

Swing to gait
Crutches move, then both legs follow

Swing through gait
Crutches move, then both legs follow

FIGURE 16–1. Crutch gaits.

- Swing-through gait, in which both crutches are moved forward, then both legs are swung through, to a position ahead of the crutches

Walkers are made of aluminum, with either wheels or rubber-tipped feet in the front, and rubber-tipped feet in the rear. Walkers are usually adjustable; they should be set up so the user's elbows are bent 20° to 30° for maximum support. The user either picks up the rear legs and rolls the walker forward or picks up the entire walker and places it forward about 18 inches to 2 feet, then steps up and into the back of the walker.

Taking Medication Correctly

The medical assistant plays an important role in managing patient medications and in educating patients about proper use of medication. The most important instructions to give patients are:

- Take all medication prescribed even if you are feeling better.
- Don't change the medication dose unless instructed by the doctor.
- Report medication side effects to the doctor.

PROCEDURE TO TEACH A PATIENT TO USE A METERED-DOSE INHALER

1. Wash hands.
2. Identify and greet the patient, and explain the procedure.
3. Open the inhaler package and demonstrate how to use it. Point out the parts and explain the use of each (mouth piece, medication bottle, plastic extender chamber/spacer if ordered).
4. Place the medication canister into the holder and shake (Fig. 16–2A).
5. Then have the patient remove the cap from the holder (Fig. 16–2B).
6. Show the patient how to fit the spacer (if used), and shake the spacer (Fig. 16–2C).
7. Coach the patient on how to hold the inhaler, push down the canister, and inhale deeply while closing the mouth with the lips firmly around mouth piece (Fig. 16–2D).
8. The medication should be inhaled deep into the patient's lungs (Fig. 16–2E).
9. Instruct the patient to remove the medication canister and rinse the holder after each use (Fig. 16–2F).

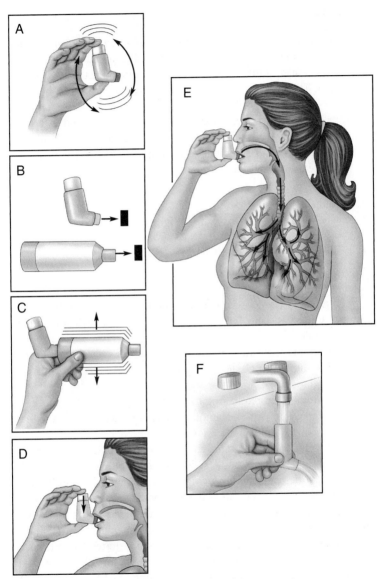

FIGURE 16–2. Steps to use a metered-dose inhaler.

Dietary Modifications

The Food Guide Pyramid, shown in Figure 16–3 (p. 205), shows the number of servings of each food group that a 175-lb man should have each day. Smaller adults and children should adjust their intake accordingly. The Food Guide Pyramid provides the pieces of a healthy diet.

Your office should have Food Guide Pyramid sheets with descriptions of the various foods at each level of the pyramid. These should be available in English and other languages commonly spoken by patients.

Restricted diets include:

- Liquid diet
- Low-calorie, low-carbohydrate, weight-loss diet
- Low-sodium diet
- Low-fat, low-cholesterol diet
- Fiber modifications

A liquid diet is necessary before certain diagnostic tests of the gastrointestinal tract and for a period of time after diarrhea or other medical problems.

Clear liquids are water, apple juice, clear broth and non-red sports drinks. Full liquids include cranberry juice and juices with pulp (orange or grapefruit).

Low-calorie diets reduce the total intake of calories. (A calorie is the unit of measure for the amount of energy needed to raise the temperature of 1 kg of water by 1°C.)

When calorie intake is more than energy needs, the extra calories are stored by the body as fat. A sedentary adult burns between 1500 and 2000 calories per day. Reducing intake below 1500 calories and increasing exercise, which burns more calories, results in weight loss.

Low-sodium diets can vary from no salt added at the table to a complete restriction on salt in cooking. Moderate salt (sodium) restriction is prescribed to control blood pressure. To reduce sodium, a patient needs to be educated about careful shopping, changing food preparation and cooking style, and eliminating salt from the table. A salt substitute may be used if approved by the physician.

It is currently recommended for all individuals that fat should comprise less than 30% of total daily caloric intake, with no more than 10% coming from saturated fats. A low-fat diet reduces fat intake even

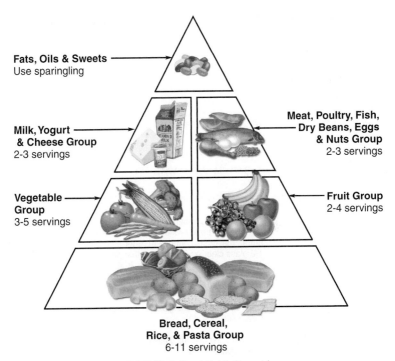

Fats, Oils & Sweets
Use sparingling

Milk, Yogurt & Cheese Group
2-3 servings

Meat, Poultry, Fish, Dry Beans, Eggs & Nuts Group
2-3 servings

Vegetable Group
3-5 servings

Fruit Group
2-4 servings

Bread, Cereal, Rice, & Pasta Group
6-11 servings

FIGURE 16–3. Food Guide Pyramid.

more severely. Patients may need instruction on foods to restrict or avoid.

A low-cholesterol diet is one that includes less than 300 mg of cholesterol intake daily. Foods high in cholesterol include liver, shellfish, egg yolk, and dairy foods (milk and cheeses). Simply reducing dietary cholesterol does not always reduce blood cholesterol enough, so some patients will need medication as well.

Fiber is the indigestible material found in plants, often composed of cellulose, which adds bulk to the diet. An increase in fiber can help reduce constipation and has been shown to be a preventive measure against colon cancer. High-fiber foods include whole grains, fruits, and most vegetables.

Some individuals with digestive diseases, such as diverticulitis, ulcerative colitis, and Crohn's disease, may have to reduce the fiber in their diet because it sometimes exacerbates symptoms.

INFORMATION FOR PATIENTS SCHEDULED FOR TESTS AT MEMORIAL HOSPITAL:

PATIENT'S NAME: _____

PROCEDURE: BARIUM ENEMA

DATE: _____

PREPARATION: CHECK IN AT OUTPATIENT REGISTRATION 15 MINUTES
                     BEFORE TEST.

BARIUM ENEMA WITH AIR

1. 12:00 NOON – LUNCH – Eat only the following:

> 1 cup of boullion soup with crackers.
> 1 chicken or turkey white meat sandwhich (no butter, mayonaise, lettuce or other additive).
> 1/2 glass clear apple juice or clear grape juice.
> 1 serving plain Jello (no cream, fruit, or other additive).
> 1 glass of skimmed or nonfat dry milk.

2. 1:00 PM   Drink at least one full glass or more of water, clear juice or soda.

3. 3:00 PM   Drink at least one full glass or more of water, clear juice or soda.

4. 4:00 PM   Drink one 11 ounce bottle of Magnesium Citrate (cold). Can be purchased from your local Pharmacy.

5. 5:00 PM – DINNER – Eat only the following:

> 1 cup of boullion soup
> 1 glass of clear apple juice or clear grape juice.
> 1 serving of plain Jello (no cream, fruit or other additive).

6. 7:00 PM   Drink at least one full glass or more of water, clear juice or soda. Take 3 biscodyl tablets (can be purchased from your local pharmacy) with at least one full glass or more of water.

7. Before Bed   Drink at least one full glass or more of water, clear juice or soda.

8.   Nothing to eat or drink after midnight.

Take 1 ounce of Milk of Magnesia after all barium studies (UGI, BE, Small Bowel) unless otherwise indicated by M.D.

FIGURE 16–4. Sample preparation sheet for a barium enema.

Preparing for Procedures

Patients need instruction prior to diagnostic procedures. This can include dietary modifications (e.g., fasting for blood tests), bowel preparation (e.g., for gastrointestinal tests), or adjustments to the time or amount of regular medication taken. Sheets containing instructions should be obtained from the facility where the test will be done because they may differ. If the appointment is made in the office, the instruction sheet can be given to the patient. Figure 16–4 is a sample instruction sheet for a barium enema. Table 16–2 identifies preparation requirements for common diagnostic tests.

TABLE 16–2
Instructions for Various Diagnostic Tests

Test	Purpose	Preparation	Instructions
Upper gastrointestinal (GI) series (barium swallow)	To visualize the esophagus, stomach, duodenum, and sometimes the small intestine; the patient swallows a flavored drink containing barium	Light evening meal the day before the test NPO after midnight	Schedule after barium enema or cholecystogram Be sure that the patient is not pregnant Increased fluids and possibly milk of magnesia after the test to help evacuate barium
Barium enema (lower GI)	To visualize the colon by introducing barium through the rectum; the patient retains the enema while placed into various positions for x-rays; air may be pumped into the colon	Clear liquid diet the day before the test, with regular fluids Laxative(s) to empty the GI tract the evening before the test NPO after midnight Enema(s) to empty the lower colon and rectum the morning of the test	Increased fluids and possibly milk of magnesia after the test to help evacuate barium Be sure that the patient is not pregnant

(continued)

TABLE 16–2
Instructions for Various Diagnostic Tests *Continued*

Test	Purpose	Preparation	Instructions
Cholecys-togram	To visualize the gall bladder and gallstones if present; ultrasound of the gallbladder is also commonly used	Fat-free evening meal the day before the test Take all tablets prescribed by MD the night before the test with 8 oz of water NPO after taking the tablets containing contrast medium Sometimes instructed to use laxative(s) and/or enemas to empty the GI tract before the test	Preparation may have to be repeated if the gallbladder cannot be seen After initial films are finished, may be instructed to eat a fatty meal and return for additional x-rays Be sure that the patient is not pregnant
Intrave-nous chol-angio-gram	To visualize the gallbladder and biliary ducts after administration of intravenous contrast medium	NPO after midnight Sometimes instructed to use laxative(s) and/or enemas to empty the GI tract before the test	Test may take several hours. Be sure that the patient is not pregnant
Pelvic ultrasound	Frequently used during pregnancy to check fetal age, position, etc.	Drink 4–6 glasses of water in the hour before the test to be sure that the bladder is full	—

TABLE 16–2			
Instructions for Various Diagnostic Tests *Continued*			
Test	*Purpose*	*Preparation*	*Instructions*
Mammo-gram	Used to identify breast cancer and other conditions of the breast	Do not wear de-odorant or pow-der on the day of the test	Previous films (if any) should be available for comparison
Magnetic resonance imaging (MRI)	Used to make an image of various body parts	Do not wear any metal objects	Patients with im-planted pace-makers or pros-theses usually cannot undergo MRI.

Preparing a Patient for Outpatient Surgery

Prior to surgery in a day-surgery facility or hospital, a patient may need to:

- Be NPO (if undergoing general anesthesia).
- Shower with a special disinfectant soap.
- Shave the area where the surgery will be performed.
- Administer an enema at home.
- Stop taking particular medications (e.g., anticoagulants).
- Arrange for transportation to and from the place where the surgery will be performed.
- Understand that valuable items should be left at home.

FOLLOW-UP CARE

Sometimes patients need to care for themselves after a diagnostic procedure or treatment.

Cast Care

After a cast has been applied, the patient should be told that:

- The extremity should be elevated.
- Ice packs should be put around the cast to reduce swelling.
- The cast should not get wet (plaster should not get wet at all, fiberglass for 48 hours to give it time to completely cure).

- Nothing should be poked under the cast to scratch an itch.
- Fingers or toes should be wiggled regularly for the first 24 hours.
- Fingers or toes should be pink and warm (white, blue, or very cold should be reported to the office).
- Drainage that stains the cast should be reported if it increases in size.

Care of Dressings and Bandages

For bandages and dressing, patients should be educated to:

- Elevate if an extremity.
- Use a sling if necessary for an arm.

  They also need to be told:

- When to return for first dressing change and other follow-up
- How to change the dressing and bandage
- What symptoms to report to the office

SOURCES FOR PATIENT-EDUCATION MATERIALS

A number of resources are available to help you put together patient teaching and to provide handouts for patients. These include:

- National organizations dealing with the particular disease or condition
- Government sources (e.g., National Institutes of Health)
- Internet

  You should develop a resource list for each type of teaching you do and frequently update it as you find new material.

Chapter 17

Office Operations

MANAGING SUPPLIES AND EQUIPMENT

At the beginning of each day, you should stock examination rooms with the amount of each supply it needs for the day. When supplies in storage run low, notify the person responsible for ordering so more can be purchased. You may be asked to order supplies, put away supplies that have been received, or inventory the central supply room to identify which supplies need to be ordered.

PROCEDURE FOR INVENTORY OF SUPPLIES

1. Obtain the inventory list, either an inventory notebook, computer file, or box of inventory cards.
2. Check all examining rooms and storage areas to find the level of inventory. Check expiration dates and dispose of supply inventory that is past date.
3. Count remaining items and write or key number in the appropriate place.
4. Check the number of items on hand against the number listed as the reorder point; if the number on hand is below or very close to the reorder point, flag the item as one that needs to be ordered.
5. Place inventory list in the proper location for follow-up and ordering.

PROCEDURE TO STOCK NEWLY ORDERED SUPPLIES

1. When an order arrives, bring it to supply closet or supply room.
2. Unpack the supplies and check what is received against the packing slip.
3. Shelve supplies, making sure to place older supplies in front of those just arrived. Check expiration dates of all old supplies to make sure they are still good.
4. Note on inventory sheet, card, or in computer how much of each supply was received. Be sure to remove any "flags" that signaled the need to order.
5. File the invoice and/or packing slip in the file for bills to be paid.

PROCEDURE TO ORDER SUPPLIES

1. Collect the list of items to be purchased (supply items that have been flagged during inventory, items that are ordered on a regular basis, or equipment and/or supplies that a doctor has requested).
2. Use either the form provided by the vendor or an office-generated form that has been approved by the vendor to place the order. It is also possible to place some orders online using a vendor's Web site.
3. List all needed supplies, noting quantity, size, color, and price.
4. Make sure you have a purchase order number for the order.
5. Total the order, including tax and shipping charges.
6. Have the purchase order signed or approved by an individual authorized to do so.
7. Mail, phone in, or fax the order, or click the *place order* button on the Web site screen.
8. Be sure to indicate in your ordering system which items were ordered, and remove any flags placed on items that needed to be ordered.
9. Place a copy (make hard copy if using a computer) in the appropriate file for pending orders.

MAINTENANCE

Always be on the lookout for equipment problems, especially those that can be dangerous. Make sure all instruments have been properly sterilized. Look for frayed wires, bent or damaged instruments, and machines that are malfunctioning.

Most pieces of medical office equipment are purchased or leased with a service contract included. Such contracts usually allow for unlimited repair calls for a specified time period. Service contracts go into effect after the manufacturer's warranty expires.

Before calling in a service technician, check the equipment thoroughly. A plug accidentally removed from a socket or a wire disconnected is often the cause of what seems to be a machine breakdown.

Make sure to conduct all routine preventive maintenance (or have a technician do so) according to manufacturer's guidelines.

Document all service calls, the reason the call was made, the response, whether there was a service charge, and any suggested follow-up.

COMPUTER SYSTEMS

After the telephone, the computer is probably the most frequently used, and possibly the most important, piece of equipment in the modern medical office. As a medical assistant, you must be familiar with computer hardware and with the particular software packages used in the office.

The individual pieces of the computer system (the hardware) are categorized by their function, as:

- Input devices, used to bring data into the computer
- Processing, in which the computer performs calculations and manipulations of data
- Storage, in which data are stored for future use
- Output devices, by which data that have been manipulated and turned into useful information (e.g., reports) are taken out of the computer

Input devices include:

- Keyboard

- Mouse
- Modem
- Scanner

Processing occurs in the central processing unit (CPU), in which there is random access memory (RAM), memory that can store information while the computer is on, and read-only memory (ROM), information that can be used but cannot be deleted. Inside the memory unit also sits a motherboard, a printed circuit board on which all of the computer's microcircuitry sits.

Every computer uses an operating system, a software program that comprises the basic commands for the computer, including how to communicate between the CPU and all of the various input and output devices. The operating system can be thought of as analogous to a human brain's basic limbic functions (heat sensation, touch, breathing, and so on).

Computers store information either on a hard drive, a unit that sits inside the computer, on an external storage unit, such as a diskette, CD-ROM, or magnetic tape. All data and information stored on the hard drive should also be routinely "backed up" onto external storage and those storage units kept outside the office so files can be reconstructed in the event of the office's devastation by fire, flood, or other occurrence. Find out how backups are handled in your office.

Output devices include:

- Monitor
- Printer
- Modem

A modem (modulator–demodulator) is both an input device and an output device. The modem translates the digital data bits in the computer into a signal that can travel over telephone wires, then retranslates it at the receiving end from telephone signals to data bits to be brought into the receiving computer.

If the operating system is analogous to the human brain's most basic functions, the higher mental processes of thinking, manipulating, computing, and sorting out relationships between items are taken into the world of the computer by application software, software that contains specific instructions about how the computer should carry out particular tasks.

The most common application software used by medical offices includes:

- Relational data base management (patient records, appointment scheduling, doctor's calendars)
- Financial management (bookkeeping, billing, check writing)
- Word processing (letters, memos, reports)
- Communication (electronic communication of bills, letters, purchase orders, patient reports).

Appendix A

Common Words and Phrases in Spanish

Do you speak English?
¿Habla Usted inglés?
ah-blah oo-s**thed** een-**glehs**

I don't understand.
No entiendo.
noh ehn-t-**yehn**-doh

My name is . . .
Me llamo . . .
meh **yah**-moh

Speak more slowly, please.
Hable más despacio, por favor.
ah-bleh mahs dehs**pahs**-yoh, pohr fah-**vohr**

Do you understand?
¿Entiende Usted?
ehn-t-**yehn**-deh oo-**stehd**

Are you allergic to anything?
¿Es Usted alérgico* a cualquier cosa?
ehs oo-**stehd** ah-**alehr**-hee-koh ah kwalk-k **yehr koh**-sah

Do you take any medications?
¿Toma medicamentos?
toh-mah meh-dee-ka-**mehn**-tos

---

*If speaking to a woman, use alérgica (ah-**alehr**-hee-ka)

You may not eat or drink anything before surgery (before the test).
No comerá o beberá nada antes de la cirugia (antes de la prueba).
no koh-meh-**rah** oh beh-beh-**rah** nah-dah **ahn**-tehs deh la see-oo-**hee**-ah
    (**ahn**-tes deh la proo-**ay**-vah)

Do you have pain?
¿Tiene dolor?
t-**yehn**-neh doh-**lohr**

Are you nauseated?
¿Siente el estómago revuelto?
s-**yehn**-teh ehl ehs-**toh**-mah-goh reh-**vwehl**-toh

Take a deep breath in, please. Exhale.
Respire profundo, por favor. Exhale.
reh-**spee**-reh proh-**foon**-doh, pohr fah-**vohr**. ehks-**ah**-leh

Don't talk, please.
No hable, por favor.
noh **ah**-bleh, pohr fah-**vohr**

I am going to give you an injection.
Le voy a poner una inyección.
leh voy a poh-**nehr** oo-nah een-yehk-s-**yohn**

I have some medications for you to take.
Tengo unas medicinas para que Usted las toma.
tehn-goh **oo**-nahs meh-dee-**see**-nahs pah-rah keh oo-**stehd** lahs **toh**-meh

How many children do you have?
¿Cuantos niños tiene Usted?
kwahn-tohs **nihn**-yos t-**yehn**-eh oo-**stehd**

Are you pregnant?
¿Está embarazada?
ehs-**tah** ehm-bahr-ah-**sah**-dah

What is your name, address, and telephone number?
¿Cuál es su nombre, dirección y teléfono?
Kwal ehs sue **nohm**-bray, dee-rehk-s-**yohn** ee teh-**lay**-foh-noh

Do you take . . . ?
¿Toma Usted . . .
toh-mah oo-**stehd**

Antibiotics?
¿Antibiótico?
ahn-tih-bee-**oh**-tih-coh

Anticoagulants?
¿Anticuagulante?
ahn-tih-koo-ah-g-oo-**lahn**-teh

Medicine for high blood pressure?
¿Medicina para la presión alta?
meh-dee-**see**-nah pah-rah lah preh-s-**yohn ahl**-tah

Antihistamines?
¿Antihistamínico?
ahn-tee-hist-ah-**meen**-ee-koh

Insulin or medicine for diabetes?
¿Insulina o medicina para la diabetes?
ihn-sue-**leen**-ah oh meh-dee-**see**-nah pah-rah lah dee-ah-**bay**-tess

Digitalis or medicine for the heart?
¿Digital o medicina para el corazón?
dee-gee-**tahl** oh meh-dee-**see**-nah pah-rah ell **koh**-rah-**sohn**

Nitroglycerin?
¿Nitroglicerina?
nee-troh-glee-seh-r-**een**-ah

Birth control pills?
¿Pastillas anticonceptivas?
pah-st-**ee**-yas ahn-tee-kon-sep-t-**ee**-vahs

Other medication?
¿Otra medicinas?
oh-trah meh-dee-**see**-nahs

Do you have or have you had any of these illnesses (conditions)?
¿Tiene o ha tenido algunas de estas condiciones (enfermidades)?
T-**yehn**-eh oh ah teh-**nee**-doh ahl-**goo**-nahs day **ehs**-tahs kon-dee-see-**yohn**-ehs (ehn-fehr-mee-**dah**-dehs)

AIDS or other conditions of the immune system?
¿SIDA o otras enfermedades immunosupresivas?
see-dah oh **oh**-trahs ehn-fehr-mee-**dah**-dehs im-**moon**-oh-sue-preh-s-**ee**-vahs

Alcohol or drug abuse?
¿Abuso del alcohol o drogas?
ah-**boo**-soh dell ahl-ko-**hohl** oh **droh**-gahs

Asthma?
¿Asma?
ahs-mah

Epilepsy?
¿Epilepcia?
eh-pih-leh-p-**see**-yah

Diabetes?
¿Diabetes?
dee-ah-**bay**-tess

Heart problems?
¿Problemas del corazón?
proh-**bleh**-mahs dehl koh-rah-**sohn**

High blood pressure or low blood pressure?
?Presion alta o presion baja?
preh-s-**yohn ahl**-tah oh preh-s-**yohn bah**-hah

Malaria?
¿Paludismo?
pah-loo-**dee**-s-moh

Persistent cough or bloody vomit?
¿Tos persistente o vomita sangre?
tohs pehr-see-s-**ten**-teh oh **voh**-mih-tah **san**-greh

Rheumatic fever?
¿Fiebre reumática?
f-**yeh**-b-reh roo-**mah**-tih-kah

Tuberculosis?
¿Tuberculosis?
too-behr-koo-**loh**-sees

Adapted from DeWit SC: *Saunders Student Nurse Planner,* Version 2. Philadelphia, W.B. Saunders, 1999; with permission.

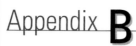

Appendix **B**

Metric System Conversions

WEIGHT EQUIVALENTS

	Metric	Apothecary
Grams (g)	*Milligrams (mg)*	*Grains (gr)*
1.0	1000	15
0.5	500	7½
0.3	300 (325)	5
0.1	100	1½
0.06	60 (64)	1
0.03	30 (32)	½
0.015	15 (16)	¼
0.010	10	⅙
0.0006	0.6	¹⁄₁₀₀
0.0004	0.4	¹⁄₁₅₀
0.0003	0.3	¹⁄₂₀₀

VOLUME EQUIVALENTS

Metric	Apothecary or Household
940 mL =	1 quart (1 quart ≈ 1L)
30 mL =	1 oz (fl ℥) = 2 Tbsp = 6 tsp
15 mL =	½ oz = 1 Tbsp = 3 tsp
5 mL =	1 tsp
4 mL =	1 fl dr (fl ʒ)
1 mL =	15 (16) minims = 15 (16) drops (gtt)

From J. Kee, and E. Hayes: *Pharmacology: A Nursing Process Approach,* 2nd ed. Philadelphia, W.B. Saunders, 1997.

Index

Note: Page numbers followed by f indicate figures; those followed by t indicate tables; those followed by b indicate boxed material.